T0020768

5-INGREDIENT COOKBOOK FOR MEN

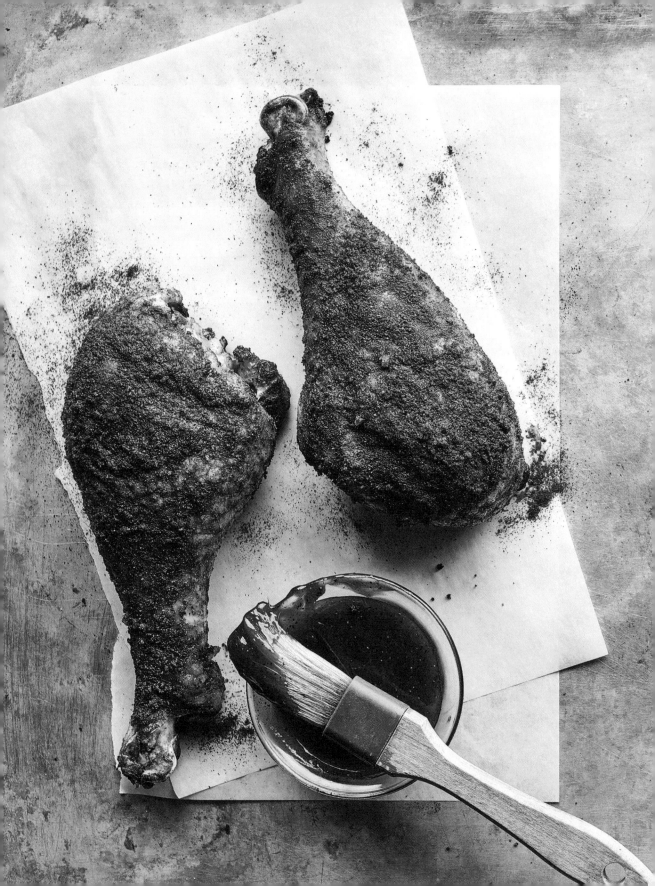

5-INGREDIENT

— COOKBOOK —

FOR MEN

WITH

BIG APPETITES

AND **LITTLE TIME**

BENJAMIN KELLY

PHOTOGRAPHY BY JOHNNY AUTRY

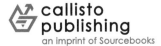

callisto
publishing
an imprint of Sourcebooks

Copyright © 2021 by Callisto Publishing LLC

Cover and internal design © 2021 by Callisto Publishing LLC

Photography © 2020 Johnny Autry, Food styling by Charlotte Autry

Illustrations: Brigantine Designs/Creative Market, Icons by Hey Rabbit, Amethyst Studio

Interior and Cover Designer: Angie Chiu

Art Producer: Megan Baggott

Editor: Gurvinder Singh Gandu

Production Editor: Rachel Taenzler

Callisto and the colophon are registered trademarks of Callisto Publishing LLC.

All rights reserved. No part of this book may be reproduced in any form or by any electronic or mechanical means including information storage and retrieval systems—except in the case of brief quotations embodied in critical articles or reviews—without permission in writing from its publisher, Sourcebooks LLC.

All brand names and product names used in this book are trademarks, registered trademarks, or trade names of their respective holders. Callisto Publishing is not associated with any product or vendor in this book.

Published by Callisto Publishing LLC C/O Sourcebooks LLC

P.O. Box 4410, Naperville, Illinois 60567-4410

(630) 961-3900

callistopublishing.com

Printed in the United States of America

VP 17

FOR MY MOM

CONTENTS

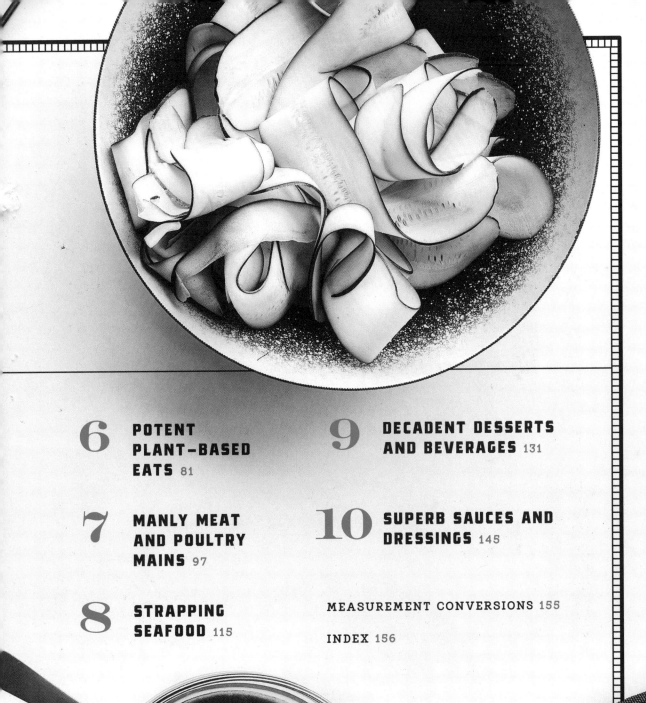

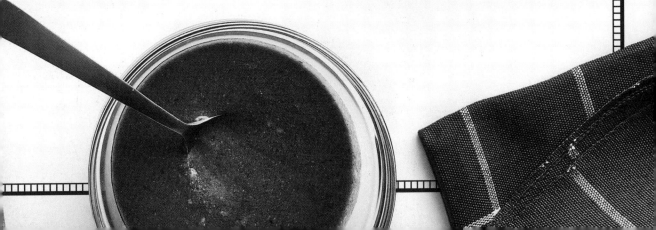

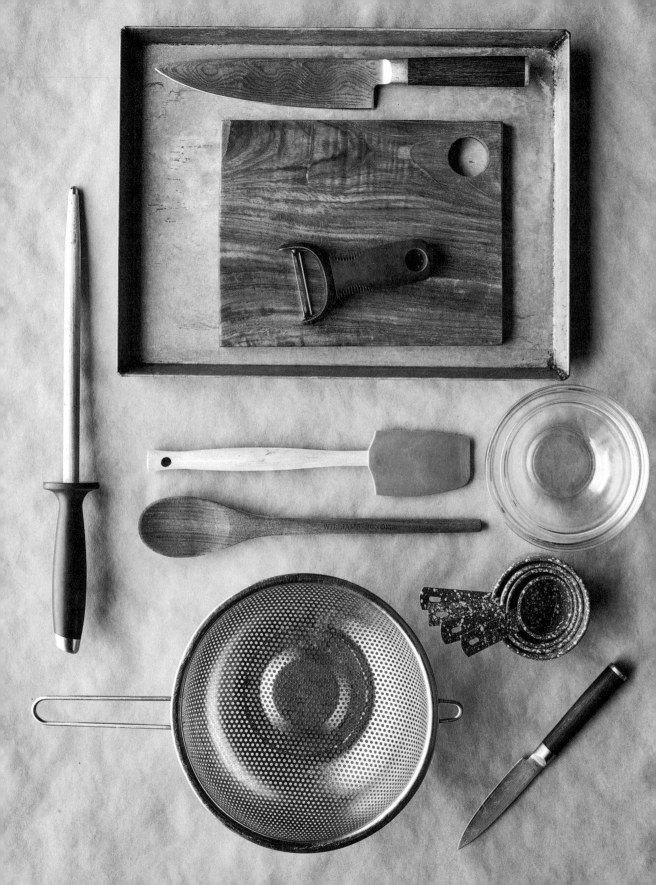

INTRODUCTION

Some of my earliest and fondest memories are of being in the kitchen cooking alongside my mother. It was those times—the smells, tastes, and sounds—that made me realize from a young age that I wanted to be a chef. Those memories still drive my love of cooking to this day.

You will find a few recipes in this book that say "Mom's"—these are my mom's actual recipes, the ones that I grew up on, the ones that I first learned to cook, and the ones that I will first teach to my son when he is old enough. My mom passed away a few years ago, but every time I cook one of her recipes, I feel connected to her. Every bite is like she's there giving me a big hug. If you take anything away from this book it should be this: Cooking is a form of connection. You connect to the ingredients you're preparing; to the people you're feeding; to the past, present, and future (you don't even need a DeLorean to do it!); and you can even find a deeper connection to yourself. (Yeah, cooking isn't all knives and fire—there are feelings here, too.)

From my mom's kitchen, I progressed to the world of professional cooking (cue the restaurant walkthrough scene from *Goodfellas*). The world of professional cooking is high-pressure, high-speed, and high-impact. It is intense at times, and the only way to get through that is to rely on the people who are in it with you. You need to be able to trust that the person beside you has your back, otherwise the whole thing falls apart. Keep that in mind as you cook from this book: You're not alone. I've got your back. We're a team and I won't let you down.

Do you remember what it was like when you first learned to ride a bike? What about when you got your first car? That sense of freedom and accomplishment that you got from those experiences can also come from learning to cook. Taking that first bite of a beautiful meal that you put the effort into cooking offers that same sense of freedom, accomplishment, and pride. You earned that meal and those feelings (yeah, I said the "F" word). You took raw ingredients and created something that is more than the sum of its parts. Make sure you allow yourself a second or two to reflect on that as you enjoy the fruits of your labor.

At first glance, five ingredients may seem a bit restrictive—I mean, what can you really do with so few ingredients? Don't worry, you'll see. But first, take a second and think back to a time when you were trying to make a decision and there were no limitations. Maybe you were trying to decide something big, like what career path to take. Or maybe it was just what you wanted to eat for dinner. If you're anything like me, you probably struggled to make a decision in those situations. There are just too many good options. On the other hand, was there a time when you had to make a decision and there were only a couple possible choices? Was that an easier decision to make? Probably. The more options we have, the harder it is to decide. In a lot of ways, cooking follows this same principle. Restricting the number of ingredients forces creativity. In other words, sometimes being put inside a box is the best way to think outside of it.

Cooking with only five ingredients means that there's less shopping, there are fewer ingredients to stock, mistakes are less likely to happen, cleanup takes less time, and cooking is quicker. Those are all good things. Like anything, cooking becomes easier with practice, but in the beginning you're going to need every advantage you can get—and limiting recipes to only five ingredients is a big advantage. As a cooking rookie, it's easy to confuse things (*was that supposed to be a teaspoon or a tablespoon?*). Keeping the ingredient lists short will help you focus on the technique and the quality of the dish rather than using all your attention to keep track of a hundred ingredients.

One thing that I want you to keep in mind as you start this journey from cooking Padawan to full-blown Jedi Master is that everyone makes mistakes. There will be days when you are faced with the decision to either eat something you cooked that didn't turn out or throw it out and start again. I still have those days sometimes. That's called learning, and it's an important part of the process. It sucks—trust me, I know—but don't beat yourself up over it. Accept the goose egg, get that dirt off your shoulder, and get back in the game.

Before we move on, I just want to give you a quick pat on the back. You picked this book up and you've read this far—that's a big step and a really important one. A former chef/mentor/current close friend once told me that, "The hardest part of traveling is buying the ticket." Well, you've bought your ticket. You've started your journey. The hardest part is over. Now the fun begins.

LET'S EAT!

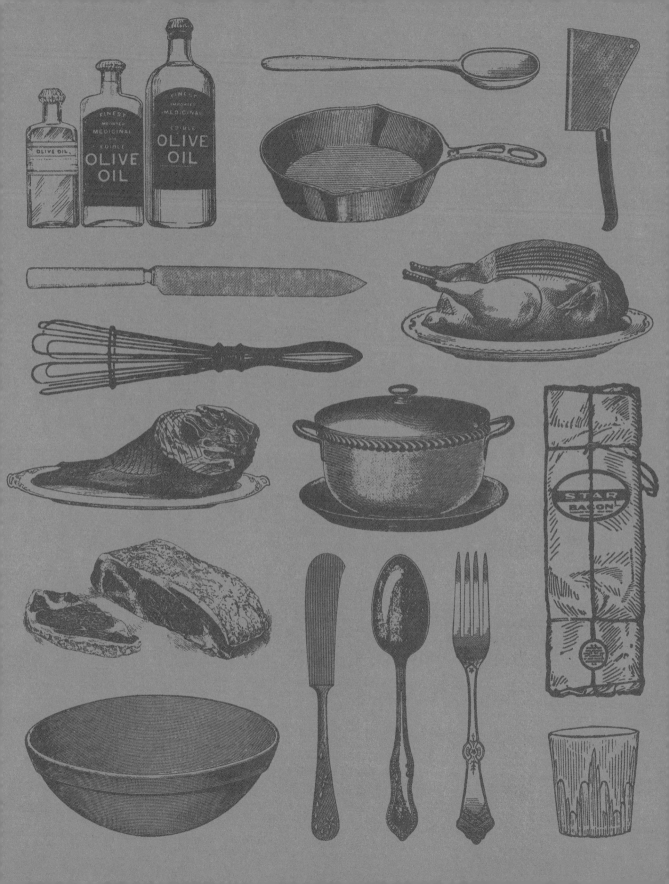

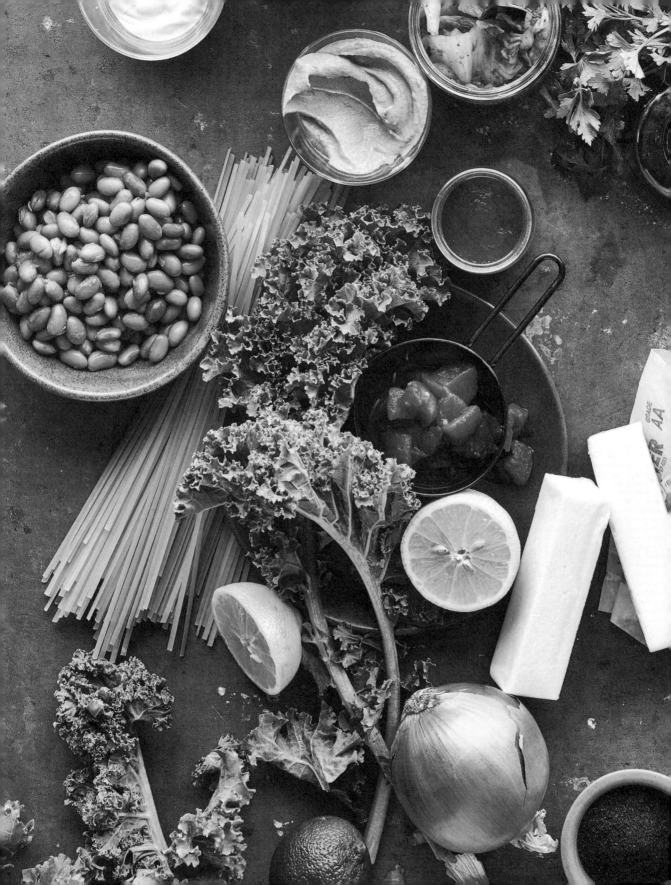

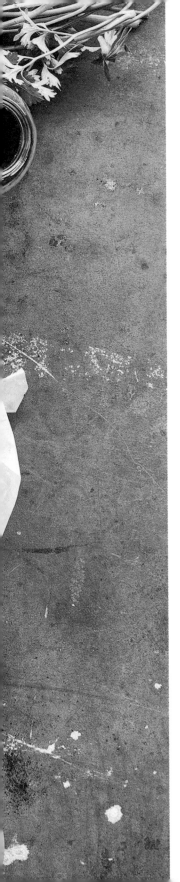

— 1 —

THE BASICS

Before you start cooking, there are some things you should know. In this first chapter, you'll get an idea of the key equipment and ingredients you should have in your kitchen. And you'll be given some basic kitchen safety principles, as well as some tips about how to navigate the grocery store. Finally, you'll get a feel for how the recipes will be laid out. Ready?

EAT LIKE A MAN

Go grab a medium onion. Seriously, I'll wait. Chances are you looked at a bag of onions and had no idea which one was a "medium" onion. What if I said go grab a baseball-size onion? Would that make more sense? That's the goal of this book: to help cooking make sense to you by using language that you understand. Yes, you have fun along the way, too. You're going to learn real skills that will make you more independent by making you better at feeding yourself. More important, you're going to cook food that you actually want to eat, while dirtying as few dishes as possible.

It is no secret that it's kind of silly to have a cookbook just for men. But for some reason, a lot of dudes think that cooking isn't masculine. This book exists to prove them wrong and to celebrate the long history of men putting meat to fire. So grab an old-fashioned, channel your inner Gordon Ramsay, and karate kick the hell out of your expectations, because cooking is one of the most masculine things that you can do and this book is going to show you why.

LESS IS MORE, MORE IS LESS

Cooking with only five ingredients allows you to see how each ingredient interacts with and complements the other because there's nothing to hide behind. Another benefit is that you learn the most valuable lesson in cooking, which most professional chefs never learn: Cooking is not about using as many ingredients as you can to make a dish taste good. It's about using as few ingredients as possible to enhance the flavor of something that already naturally tastes great.

STOCKING YOUR KITCHEN FOR 5-INGREDIENT COOKING

One of the most important parts of cooking is being prepared. That means having everything on hand and ready to go when you need it. This section is all about making sure you have the ingredients that you'll need when it comes time to get cooking. The following lists are broken down into sections of your kitchen, including the fridge, freezer, spice rack, and so on. Don't go out and buy all of this stuff at once, but keep in mind that these are all good things to have on hand, especially when cooking from this book.

THE FRIDGE

CONDIMENTS: Cooking with only five ingredients means that, whenever possible, the ingredients you're using need to pull double duty. Condiments like mustard, mayonnaise, ketchup, sriracha, kimchi, pickles, and sambal oelek are fantastic for this purpose.

GREENS: Leafy greens like lettuce, kale, and spinach can add a healthy boost to smoothies or pasta, and make a great base for salads.

FRESH HERBS: Cilantro, parsley, rosemary, and thyme all add loads of flavor to even the simplest dishes and can turn an okay recipe into a great one.

SALTED BUTTER: Butter can be salted or unsalted. The salt adds flavor but also acts as a preservative, which means the butter you buy (and it is expensive) will last longer. For both of those reasons, all the butter used in this book is salted.

FRESH VEGETABLES: Carrots, celery, asparagus, broccoli, and cauliflower should be kept in the crisper drawer of your refrigerator to maximize their shelf life.

MILK AND CREAM: It's best to use whole milk (3.25 percent milk fat) when cooking. Milk is an emulsion of fat suspended in water, so the higher fat content of whole milk makes this emulsion more stable. You just got scienced!

CHEESES: Cheddar, Monterey Jack, and Parmesan are good to eat on their own, but can also add a lot of flavor to simple dishes.

THE FREEZER

PUFF PASTRY: This is the perfect go-to for quick desserts or fancy appetizers. Keep a box in the freezer for when a sweet craving hits you.

FROZEN VEGETABLES: They sometimes get a bad rap, but they're picked at the height of their growing season and frozen within hours. Frozen peas, green beans, and vegetable medley are fantastic to add to dishes or used as a quick side dish.

FROZEN FRUITS: Mango, strawberry, banana, and blueberry are great to add to smoothies or desserts.

MEAT, POULTRY, AND FISH: If you're a sucker for a bargain, buy meat, poultry, and fish in family packs, break them into smaller portions, and freeze them.

LEFTOVER SOUPS AND CASSEROLES: These can be frozen and then reheated for a quick meal, so it's a good idea to make extras for this purpose.

THE PANTRY

GARLIC: A great way to add a punch of flavor with only a small amount. Buy it by the bulb and store it in a cool, dry place.

ONIONS: One of those ubiquitous kitchen items, onions go in just about everything. Always have at least a few around and keep them in a cool, dark place.

POTATOES: Like onions, they should be kept in a cool, dark place. I suggest keeping a few all-purpose potatoes on hand such as russet. Buy specialty potatoes only when you need them.

LEMONS AND LIMES: These citrus fruits add a splash of acid and flavor to many dishes. Have a couple on hand and use them often.

ALCOHOL: Not just for drinking, wine, whiskey, and tequila are used in some recipes in this book. If you'd prefer not to use alcohol, you can substitute it with chicken stock in most recipes.

THE SPICE RACK

BLACK PEPPER: If you have a pepper grinder, great! You will get more flavor from freshly ground pepper. But pre-ground pepper is fine.

KOSHER OR SEA SALT: These have better flavor than iodized table salt and give you more control over your seasoning.

DRIED OREGANO, THYME, SAGE, AND ROSEMARY: These herbs add loads of flavor to soups and sauces. Dried store longer than fresh herbs but lack some of the upfront flavor.

SPICE BLENDS: A great way to pack in the flavor without having a pile of ingredients on hand. Recommended spice blends include chili powder, curry powder, garam masala, poultry seasoning, and Cajun seasoning. These can be found at most grocery stores.

CAYENNE PEPPER AND RED PEPPER FLAKES: Add a little spice to dishes.

CUMIN AND CORIANDER: These ground spices provide lots of flavor to both Mexican and Indian dishes.

CANNED GOODS

CANNED BEANS AND CHICKPEAS: They might take up a lot of space in the cupboard, but these are fantastic to have on hand as they're much quicker to use than dried versions. If time is of the essence, canned beans are the way to go.

CREAM-STYLE CORN: This is the key ingredient in two of my mom's recipes: Mom's Shepherd's Pie (page 98) and Bacon and Corn Chowder (page 34). It also makes a quick side dish for pork chops.

CANNED TOMATOES: Whether crushed, whole, or pureed, canned tomatoes are used in soups, sauces, and casseroles. It's a good idea to have a few extra in the cupboard because they always come in handy.

CHICKEN AND BEEF STOCK: Both can be used in place of water in most recipes to add more flavor. Beef stock is great for beef dishes while chicken stock can be used for almost anything.

DRY GOODS

OLIVE OIL: Great for a lot of things, but not all things. Grapeseed, corn, and canola oils are good neutral-flavored alternatives.

CIDER, RED WINE, RICE, AND DISTILLED WHITE VINEGAR: Use these to make salad dressing, barbecue sauce, and more. Although it's best to use the vinegar specified in the recipe, you can often substitute another type. Just note that the substitution will affect the flavor of your dish.

DRIED BEANS, LENTILS, AND CORNMEAL: Dried beans are more economical than canned ones but must be soaked overnight before use.

BASMATI, STICKY (SUSHI), AND ARBORIO RICE: Basmati is a great all-purpose rice, sticky rice is perfect for fried rice, and Arborio is used for risotto.

DRIED PASTA: This makes a quick meal or hearty side dish. Have a few different shapes of dried pasta around and use them interchangeably.

NAVIGATING THE GROCERY STORE

The grocery store is out to get you, man. Everything you see, smell, and hear in the grocery store has been meticulously curated to make you part with as much of your hard-earned cash as possible. Seriously, it's true. Have you ever noticed that the more time you spend in the store, the more money you spend? That's not an accident. They make you look like a jabroni! Here are some tips to prevent that from happening again.

SHOPPING TIPS

MAKE A LIST: Going to the grocery store without a shopping list is like fighting Cobra Kai without waxing on and off first. Make a list, check it twice, spend less money, feels so nice.

BUY IN BULK WHEN IT MAKES SENSE: Buying in bulk can save you money, but it's a good way to waste money, too. Buy things in bulk that you will eat in a reasonable amount of time.

NEVER GO TO THE GROCERY STORE HUNGRY: When you're hungry, everything looks good, and everything that looks good goes into the cart. Eat before you go.

GO AROUND THE OUTSIDE: The outside aisles of the grocery store are where the fresh vegetables, bread, meat, milk, and eggs are. Only go to the inside aisles for things like canned goods, international foods, and dried goods.

SHOP ONCE A WEEK: The more often you shop, the more money you will spend. Plan your meals, make your list, and only shop once a week. You will save time and money.

DON'T F*CK IT UP 101

You know how people say that you can't make an omelet without breaking a few eggs? Well, today you're the egg. You might get a little broken. The kitchen can be a dangerous place, and accidents happen. Luckily, Danger is your middle name and you aren't scared of a little burn or cut. Of course, there's no point in taking unnecessary risks. In this section, we're going to take a minute or two to talk about kitchen safety—like how to hold a knife properly so you don't lose a finger, and how to make sure you don't give yourself or anyone else food poisoning.

Keep in mind that everyone makes mistakes. I still burn myself from time to time. It happens. But the goal is to limit accidents as much as possible. The best way to do that is to follow basic kitchen-safety principles.

KITCHEN SAFETY

Kitchen safety goes beyond not pouring boiling water all over yourself or catching your oven mitt on fire. It also includes proper food handling, so that you don't make anyone sick. I'm not going to tell you how to live your life, but I'm pretty confident that you do not want to make anyone sick.

At the end of the day, most accidents and food poisoning can be avoided. Here are five key rules for kitchen safety that you should follow:

RAW MEATS: These should not be left at room temperature for more than 1 hour. Bacteria will grow exponentially after that time.

COOKED FOOD: Never leave it at room temperature for more than 2 hours.

THAWING FOOD: Do this in the fridge overnight, in the microwave on the defrost setting, or under cold running water. Never thaw foods by letting them sit at room temperature.

MINIMUM INTERNAL TEMPERATURE: Most foods should be heated to a minimum internal temperature of 165°F. Check your government health board for other recommended cooking temperatures.

FIRE SAFETY: You should have a basic understanding of fire safety and how to properly deal with different types of fires. Always call 911 if there is a fire.

KNIFE SKILLS

Having good knife skills means that your knife never goes anywhere that you don't want it to. When you played Little League, the coach would tell you to choke up on the bat, right? He meant to hold the bat higher on the handle to gain more control. Same goes for a knife. The higher on the handle you hold, the more control you have.

Here are five key knife skills you should master:

GUIDE THE KNIFE: Rest the side of the knife blade against the back of the fingers on the hand that isn't holding the knife—this is the guide hand. The fingertips of your guide hand should be holding the food you are cutting.

THE TRAIN KEEPS A ROLLIN': You know how an old timey train engine has that piece of metal that connects the front and back wheels? Imagine that's your knife when you are cutting. Rather than your knife going straight up and down, keep the tip of the knife on the cutting board and use the same motion as the wheel-holding metal thing.

TAKE YOUR TIME CUTTING: Professional chefs can cut things very fast. You are not a professional chef. Take your time and keep your fingers.

LEARN THE CUTS: Learning what a julienne and different sizes of dice or cubes are, and how to cut them, will help you cut quicker and more accurately.

KEEP THINGS ORDERLY: When cutting food, keep it all the same size as best you can. Big and small pieces of food are going to cook at different rates, leading to some being overcooked and some being undercooked.

KEEP IT CLEAN

The messier your kitchen is, the harder it is to stay organized and tidy. Here are a few tips that will help you keep the kitchen clean and organized as you go:

READY THE SINK: Fill it with hot, soapy water when you start cooking, so you can quickly wash dishes as you go and avoid a giant mess at the end.

TIME TO LEAN, TIME TO CLEAN: Take advantage of any downtime to wipe the counters and your cutting board. The cleaner you keep things, the easier it will be to cook.

HAVE A WASTE BOWL: Rather than reaching down to the garbage can or compost bin every few minutes, have a trash bowl on the counter for quicker cleanup.

BE PREPARED: Before you start cooking, go through the recipe and get all the food and equipment organized and ready to go. This will save you a lot of time later.

CLEAN THE KITCHEN WHEN YOU ARE DONE EATING: It's hard to get motivated to finish up the last few dishes after dinner. You ate a great meal, you're relaxed, and you don't want to ruin that by cleaning. But it's worth it to just have it done and not have to worry about it in the morning.

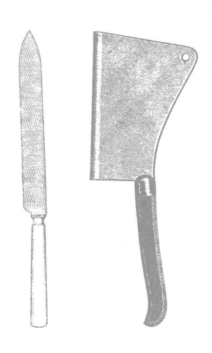

THINGS YOU NEED IN A KITCHEN THAT AREN'T A MICROWAVE

If you're building a house, you're going to need a hammer and a saw. To cook a meal, you're going to need some tools, too. Here's what to equip yourself with:

- ☐ **A CHEF'S KNIFE:** Look for a 9- or 10-inch knife that's comfortable to hold and has a sturdy blade that runs the whole length of the handle ($25 to $100 is more than enough to spend).

- ☐ **A PARING KNIFE** for small cutting tasks

- ☐ **AN INEXPENSIVE KNIFE SHARPENER:** "You're not the sharpest knife in the drawer" is an insult for a reason—dull knives are bad.

- ☐ **3 WOODEN SPOONS**

- ☐ **A SPATULA** (the egg flipper kind)

- ☐ **A RUBBER SPATULA** for scraping the sides of bowls

- ☐ **A SET OF MIXING BOWLS**

- ☐ **A SET OF GOOD-QUALITY POTS:** Look for stainless steel with a heavy bottom and a solid handle.

- ☐ **A SIEVE**

- ☐ **3 BAKING SHEETS:** Get either sheet pans—which have rimmed edges to catch juices—or unrimmed baking sheets, sometimes called cookie sheets.

- ☐ **A VEGETABLE PEELER**

- ☐ **MEASURING CUPS AND SPOONS**

- ☐ **A CUTTING BOARD**

ABOUT THE RECIPES

The goal of this book is for you to succeed at cooking. All the recipes have been designed with that in mind. You won't find anything in here that will require advanced culinary skills or knowledge. What you will find are a bunch of five-ingredient recipes for delicious food worth making.

BASE INGREDIENTS

The thing that makes a good cookbook is whether or not you want to cook and eat the recipes it contains. This cookbook is designed to be one that you return to and use again and again. However, to create crave-able dishes with only five ingredients, there will be a few concessions. Although you can do a lot with only five ingredients, there are obvious limitations. For one thing, there are four absolutely essential base ingredients that **will not** be counted toward the five ingredients. They are:

- SALT
- PEPPER
- OIL/COOKING SPRAY
- WATER

We'll assume that you have these already. (The reality is that if these base items were counted toward the 5-ingredient threshold, it would be nearly impossible to create recipes that were actually interesting and flavorful and that you'd actually want to eat.)

To make it easier to tell the base ingredients apart from the actual ingredients, the latter are highlighted in **bold** on each recipe page.

To keep the ingredient lists short, some of the recipes are cut down to their bare bones. You can cook and eat them as they are, and you will enjoy them. However, these cut-down recipes will often have suggestions for additional ingredients that can take a really good recipe and make it a great one.

✳ **A NOTE ON STICKY RICE**
Some recipes call for "sticky rice," a starchy short-grained rice variety that is used to make sushi, among other things. In grocery stores, it will be labeled either sushi rice or sticky rice. Depending on the brand, the ratio of water to rice and the cooking time may vary. That said, generally speaking, the ratio is 3:4, which translates to 1 cup of rice to 1⅓ cups of water. Rinse the rice in cold water until the water runs clear. Drain it well, then put it in a medium pot with the measured water. Bring the water to a boil, stirring the rice once in a while to make sure it doesn't stick. Once it starts to boil, turn the heat to low, put a lid on the pot, and let it simmer for 21 minutes. Take the cooked rice off the heat and let it sit for 5 minutes, then fluff it with a fork.

TIPS

Many of the recipes have tips, including suggested ingredient additions, tips about prep, possible swaps, and a variety of other things. Here are the tips you will find:

FLAVOR BOOST: Suggestions for adding to the base ingredients to make a recipe more substantial and/or to take it in a different flavor direction.

PREP TIP: How to prepare an ingredient more efficiently.

SUBSTITUTION TIP: How to replace a potentially hard to find ingredient with an easier alternative.

INGREDIENT TIP: Information on an ingredient, such as what it is, where to find it, or how it works in the recipe.

STORAGE TIP: How to store ingredients that you make separately for use in other recipes, such as dressings and seasoning sauces, or recipes that you make a lot of at once for future use, such as sausage patties.

LABELS

Along with tips, recipes will also include labels that will help you navigate the book. If you're looking for a quick meal, look for recipes labeled 30-Minute. Or, if you're cooking for a friend, look for the Easy to Double label. See the full list below.

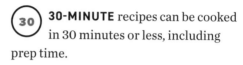 **30-MINUTE** recipes can be cooked in 30 minutes or less, including prep time.

DF **DAIRY-FREE** recipes do not contain any form of dairy (this includes butter).

x2 **EASY TO DOUBLE** recipes are great if you have a friend coming over for dinner, you're going to a potluck, or you want to make some extra food to have in the freezer.

GF **GLUTEN-FREE** recipes do not contain any products with gluten (such as wheat, barley, rye, and their derivatives) and are perfect for those with a gluten sensitivity.

OP **ONE-POT/ONE-PAN** recipes are cooked in one pot, skillet, baking dish, or other cooking vessel. You may also need a bowl or two to help with prep.

VG **VEGETARIAN** recipes do not contain any meat, poultry, or seafood.

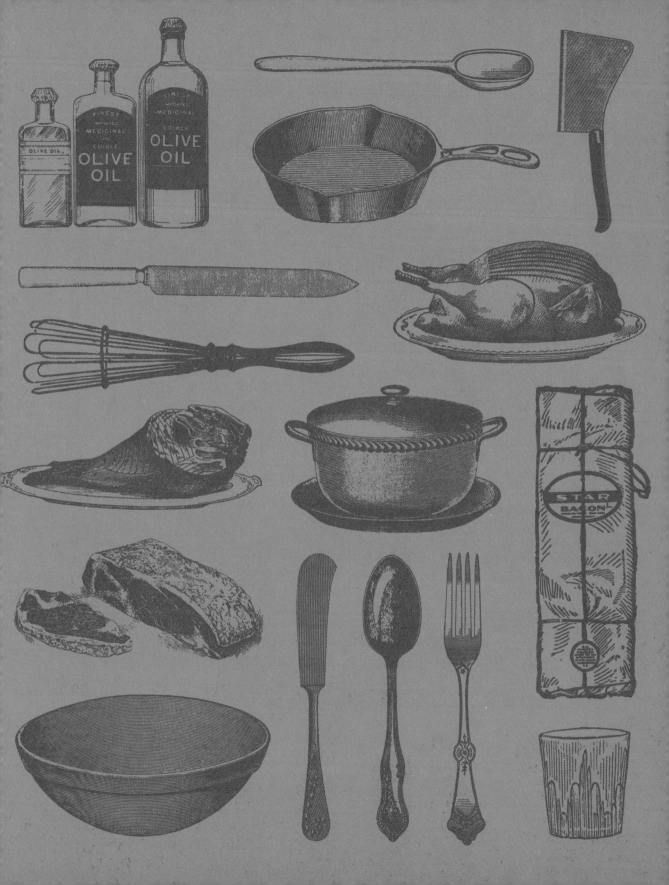

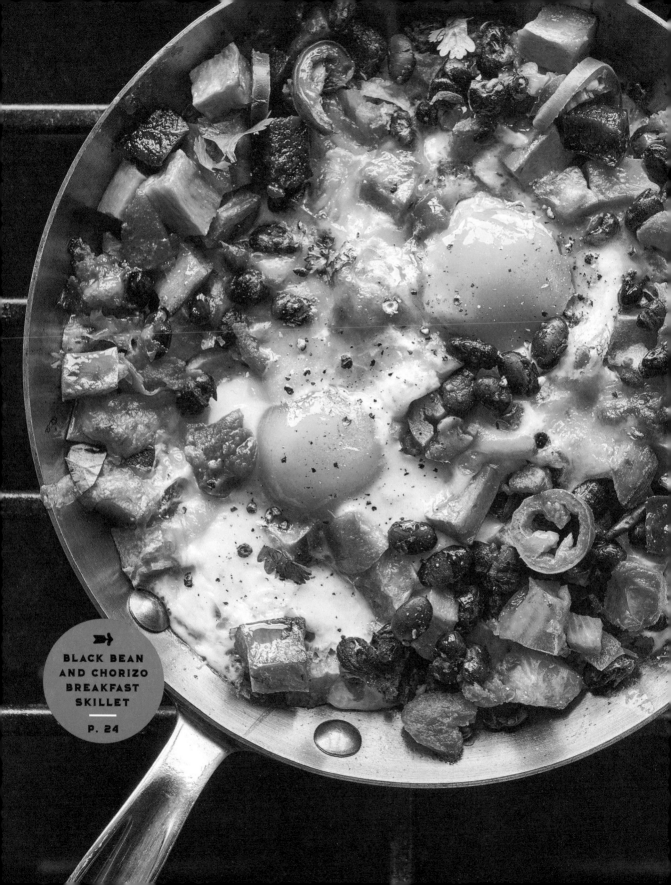

➤

BLACK BEAN
AND CHORIZO
BREAKFAST
SKILLET

P. 24

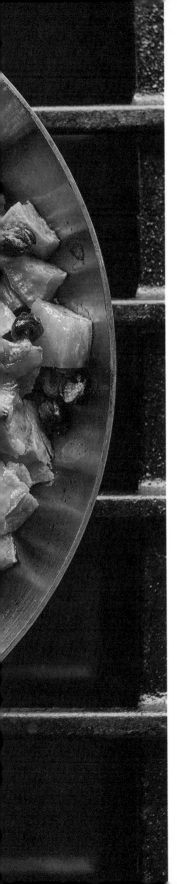

— 2 —

BURLY BREAKFASTS

5-INGREDIENT GRANOLA

MAKES: 4 cups   **PREP TIME:** 5 minutes, plus 2 hours to cool   **COOK TIME:** 30 minutes

While granola makes for an ideal breakfast, as evident by this recipe, it can also be a delicious snack, a great addition to salads, and so much more. It's best to use old-fashioned rolled oats in this recipe over quick oats because they will absorb less moisture and maintain their structure, giving the finished granola a better texture.

4 tablespoons (½ stick) salted butter, melted

¼ cup packed light brown sugar

¼ cup honey

1 cup old-fashioned rolled oats (certified gluten-free, if needed)

1 cup mixed nuts and seeds

1. Preheat the oven to 300°F. Line a sheet pan with parchment paper.

2. In a large bowl, combine the melted butter, brown sugar, and honey. Add the oats and nuts.

3. Spread the mixture onto the lined pan. Transfer to the oven and bake the granola for 30 minutes, giving it a stir every 10 minutes or so.

4. Let the mixture cool for 2 hours at room temperature, then put it into an airtight container.

✴ FLAVOR BOOST: The greater variety of seeds and nuts that you use in the granola, the better it will be. You can also mix dried fruit like cranberries or raisins into the granola once it comes out of the oven.

Per serving (½ cup): Calories: 242; Total Fat: 16g; Saturated Fat: 5g; Protein: 5g; Total Carbohydrates: 24g; Fiber: 2g; Sugar: 14g; Cholesterol: 15mg

NOT YOUR GRANDMA'S PORRIDGE

    (30) (x2) (GF) (OP) (VG)

SERVES: 2   **PREP TIME:** 5 minutes   **COOK TIME:** 10 minutes

Porridge can often seem like this boring thing that your grandparents eat, but it doesn't have to be. I mean, ancient Roman soldiers ate porridge almost every day and you wouldn't want to mess with them. You can add all kinds of fresh and dried fruit, nuts, and seeds to this porridge to make it a special breakfast item that you return to day after day.

2 cups water

¼ teaspoon ground cinnamon

2 tablespoons light brown sugar

Pinch of salt

¼ cup raisins

1 cup old-fashioned rolled oats (look for gluten-free if needed)

2 tablespoons butter, divided

1. In a medium pot, combine the water, cinnamon, brown sugar, salt, and raisins and bring to a boil.

2. Using a wooden spoon, stir the oats into the boiling water, then reduce the heat to medium-low and continue stirring for about 10 minutes, or until oats are soft and most of the water has been absorbed.

3. Stir 1 tablespoon of butter into the porridge. Scoop the porridge into two bowls, and top with the remaining 1 tablespoon of butter.

FLAVOR BOOST: For a little more kick, soak the raisins in ½ cup whiskey or brandy overnight.

Per serving: Calories: 341; Total Fat: 15g; Saturated Fat: 8g; Protein: 6g; Total Carbohydrates: 51g; Fiber: 5g; Sugar: 22g; Cholesterol: 31mg

FRITTATA BASE

MAKES: 2 cups   **PREP TIME:** 5 minutes

A frittata is like a baked omelet or a crustless quiche, but this frittata base, as you will see, can be used for so much more. Consider this recipe a blank canvas upon which you can paint your culinary masterpiece in the style of the great masters Leonardo, Michelangelo, Raphael, and Donatello.

4 large eggs
½ cup whole milk
½ cup heavy cream
¼ teaspoon salt

1. In a medium bowl, beat the eggs with a whisk until the whites and yolks are fully combined.

2. Whisk in the milk, cream, and salt until the mixture is uniform in color and texture.

3. Use the frittata base according to the specific recipe or store in the fridge for up to 3 days for later use.

Per serving (1 cup): Calories: 395; Total Fat: 34g; Saturated Fat: 18g; Protein: 16g; Total Carbohydrates: 6g; Fiber: 0g; Sugar: 6g; Cholesterol: 446mg

CHEESY MUSHROOM FRITTATA

SERVES: 2   **PREP TIME:** 5 minutes   **COOK TIME:** 15 minutes

In the name of variety, here's a more amped up version of the classic frittata that uses our base recipe from page 16. You can use any kind of mushrooms you'd like for this. I prefer a combination of cremini, oyster, and lion's mane mushrooms, but use whatever you prefer.

1 tablespoon salted butter

1 cup sliced mushrooms

Salt

Freshly ground black pepper

¼ teaspoon dried thyme

Frittata Base (page 16)

¼ cup grated cheddar cheese, divided

1. Preheat the oven to 350°F.

2. Heat a medium ovenproof nonstick skillet over medium-high heat. Add the butter and mushrooms, season with salt and pepper, and cook for about 3 minutes.

3. Add the thyme and cook for 1 more minute, then add the frittata base. Stir and cook for 30 seconds, then stir in half the cheddar. Sprinkle the rest of the cheddar on top.

4. Transfer to the oven and bake for 10 minutes. Check the doneness of the frittata by giving the pan a little shake. If the center is solid, it's ready.

5. Remove from the oven, put a plate upside down on top of it, and flip so the frittata comes out onto the plate.

✱ INGREDIENT TIP: You can put almost anything in a frittata, but avoid wet ingredients like zucchini or diced tomatoes (use whole cherry or grape tomatoes instead).

Per serving: Calories: 510; Total Fat: 45g; Saturated Fat: 24g; Protein: 21g; Total Carbohydrates: 7g; Fiber: <1g; Sugar: 7g; Cholesterol: 476mg

GRAB AND GO FRITTATA CUPS

MAKES: 12 frittata cups   **PREP TIME:** 5 minutes   **COOK TIME:** 35 minutes

In case you're really getting into frittatas now, here's a more portable take on the dish. Breakfast is the most important meal of the day—it's also the one that most often gets forgotten. You've got a lot going on in your life, but don't let breakfast slip. Make these Grab and Go Frittata Cups ahead and grab them on your way out the door. If you're a chronic over-sleeper or snooze-button hitter, these are the thing for you.

---

6 slices bacon, diced

½ cup diced onion

Frittata Base (page 16)

½ cup grated cheddar cheese

---

1. Preheat the oven to 350°F.

2. Put the bacon in a medium skillet and set it over medium heat. Let the bacon slowly heat up and cook for 7 to 8 minutes, until it starts to brown around the edges. Once the bacon starts to brown, add the onion and cook for another 5 minutes.

3. Drain the excess fat out of the pan into a small bowl or ramekin. Brush a 12-cup muffin tin with the bacon fat, then divide the onion and bacon mixture among the holes.

4. Divide the frittata base evenly among the 12 cups. Add the cheddar and stir with the handle of a spoon.

5. Bake the egg cups for 15 to 20 minutes, until the centers of the cups no longer jiggle when gently shaken.

6. Eat the muffin cups hot or cold.

   ❋ **STORAGE TIP:** Keep the muffin cups in a zip-top bag or airtight container in the fridge for up to 4 days.

Per serving (1 frittata cup): Calories: 105; Total Fat: 9g; Saturated Fat: 4g; Protein: 5g; Total Carbohydrates: 2g; Fiber: <1g; Sugar: 1g; Cholesterol: 83mg

MAPLE-BACON FRENCH TOAST

SERVES: 2   **PREP TIME:** 5 minutes   **COOK TIME:** 15 minutes

In France, French toast is called *pain perdu,* meaning "lost bread." It's called that because French toast is traditionally made with day-old, stale bread that is brought back to life by soaking it in an egg-and-milk mixture and then cooking it. This recipe is very calorie dense and should be eaten with caution. You've been warned.

4 slices (1 inch thick) sourdough bread, left
　　on the counter to dry overnight
Frittata Base (page 16)
1 tablespoon canola or corn oil
4 slices bacon, diced
¼ cup pecans
½ cup maple syrup

1. Preheat the oven to 350°F.

2. Dip the bread in the frittata base and let it soak for about 1 minute.

3. In a large skillet, heat the oil over medium-high heat. Shake any excess egg mixture off the bread, put the bread in the pan, and cook for 2 to 3 minutes per side, until the bread turns golden brown. Arrange on a baking sheet and transfer to the oven for about 10 minutes.

4. Put the bacon in the skillet and cook it until crispy, about 4 to 5 minutes. Add the pecans and maple syrup to the pan, boil for 1 minute, then remove from the heat.

5. Take the French toast out of the oven, put it on two plates, and pour the maple-bacon syrup over the top.

✳ FLAVOR BOOST: To kick the flavor up a notch, add ¼ cup bourbon or brandy to the bacon pan before adding the maple syrup and cook for 1 minute.

Per serving: Calories: 1,122; Total Fat: 65g; Saturated Fat: 23g; Protein: 32g; Total Carbohydrates: 105g; Fiber: 3g; Sugar: 58g; Cholesterol: 462mg

BANANA CHOCOLATE CHIP BREAD PUDDING CUPS

MAKES: 12 pudding cups **PREP TIME:** 10 minutes, plus 5 minutes to cool
COOK TIME: 25 minutes

Who says breakfast has to be boring? These "I'm a grown-ass man, I'll eat what I want" banana chocolate chip bread pudding cups will make you feel like a kid eating sugary cereal and watching Saturday morning cartoons.

Cooking spray
2 ripe bananas
1 cup sugar
Frittata Base (page 16)
4 cups diced stale sourdough bread
1 cup chocolate chips

1. Preheat the oven to 350°F. Mist 12 cups of a muffin tin with cooking spray and line the cups with paper liners.

2. In a large bowl, mash the bananas. Whisk in the sugar and frittata base. Add the bread and let it sit for 5 minutes.

3. Stir in the chocolate chips. Spoon the bread mixture into the 12 muffin cups.

4. Transfer to the oven and bake for 22 to 25 minutes, until the bread pudding cups are lightly browned and don't jiggle when you shake them.

5. Let the bread pudding cool for 5 minutes in the pan, then remove them from the tin. Cool completely before storing in the fridge.

Per serving (1 pudding cup): Calories: 261; Total Fat: 11g; Saturated Fat: 6g; Protein: 5g; Total Carbohydrates: 37g; Fiber: 1.5g; Sugar: 28g; Cholesterol: 78mg

HOMEMADE TURKEY SAUSAGE PATTIES

SERVES: 6 **PREP TIME:** 10 minutes **COOK TIME:** 20 minutes

Do you love sausage but hate clogged arteries? These homemade turkey sausage patties solve that problem. They're loaded with flavor, but have way less fat and cholesterol than regular sausages. Because they're fully cooked, they're a great option for a quick breakfast. Eat them with fried eggs, as a breakfast sandwich, or even in a breakfast skillet.

---

1 pound ground turkey

2 garlic cloves, minced

1 teaspoon poultry seasoning

¾ teaspoon salt

¼ teaspoon cayenne pepper

¼ teaspoon freshly ground black pepper

⅛ teaspoon ground cinnamon

1 teaspoon canola or corn oil

---

1. Preheat the oven to 375°F. Line a baking sheet with parchment paper or aluminum foil.

2. In a medium bowl, combine the turkey, garlic, poultry seasoning, salt, cayenne, black pepper, and cinnamon and mix well.

3. Divide the turkey mixture into 6 even portions and roll into balls. Press the balls into patties about ⅛ inch thick and place on the lined baking sheet.

4. Bake the sausage patties for 12 minutes.

5. Heat a medium skillet over medium-high heat. Add the oil and sear the turkey sausage patties for about 3 minutes per side, or until browned.

✱ STORAGE TIP: As you'll have more patties than you'll likely want to eat in a single sitting, store the leftovers in the fridge in an airtight container for up to 3 days. For longer storage, place in resealable bag and freeze. Let the patties cool before storing. When ready to reuse, simply reheat in microwave.

Per serving (1 patty): Calories: 139; Total Fat: 10g; Saturated Fat: 3g; Protein: 13g; Total Carbohydrates: 1g; Fiber: <1g; Sugar: 0g; Cholesterol: 59mg

KICK-ASS TURKEY SAUSAGE BREAKFAST SANDWICH

SERVES: 1   **PREP TIME:** 2 minutes   **COOK TIME:** 6 minutes

If you need a quick breakfast, nothing beats a breakfast sandwich. Turkey and Swiss make a classic combination that will help you start your day off right.

1 teaspoon canola oil
1 Homemade Turkey Sausage Patty (page 21)
1 large egg
1 English muffin
1 slice Swiss cheese
2 leaves iceberg lettuce

1. Warm a medium skillet over medium heat. Add the oil along with the sausage patty. Crack the egg into the pan alongside the sausage and cook the sausage for about 3 minutes per side, or until browned on both sides and hot in the middle. Cook the egg to your preferred doneness. Keep in mind that a runny yolk is like extra sauce for the sandwich.

2. While the sausage and egg are cooking, toast the English muffin.

3. Once the sausage is heated and browned, put it on the English muffin. Top the sausage with the cheese, egg, lettuce, and the other half of the English muffin.

✳ **FLAVOR BOOST:** Make the sandwich more substantial by adding tomato and avocado. Or, to take this in a different direction, mix together 1 teaspoon cranberry sauce and 2 tablespoons mayonnaise and spread on the English muffin.

Per serving: Calories: 501; Total Fat: 31g; Saturated Fat: 9g; Protein: 29g; Total Carbohydrates: 27g; Fiber: 2g; Sugar: 3g; Cholesterol: 243mg

QUICK AND EASY BREAKFAST BURRITO

SERVES: 1   **PREP TIME:** 10 minutes   **COOK TIME:** 15 minutes

This burrito makes a hearty and filling breakfast for those days when you wake up feeling a little empty and need a boost. Using homemade turkey sausage instead of pork sausage or bacon makes this burrito extra tasty, and maybe even a little healthy.

1 Homemade Turkey Sausage Patty (page 21)

1 teaspoon canola oil

¼ cup black bean salsa, homemade (page 49) or store-bought

2 large eggs, beaten

2 tablespoons grated cheddar cheese

1 (12-inch) whole wheat tortilla

1. Break the sausage patty into 1-inch pieces.

2. Warm a nonstick medium skillet over medium heat. Add the oil and the sausage and brown the sausage. Add the salsa and cook for another minute.

3. Pour the eggs into the pan and stir for 1 minute. Add the cheddar and cook until the eggs are cooked, about 2 minutes.

4. Put the egg and sausage mixture in the center of the tortilla and fold the bottom third of the tortilla up and over the mixture. Fold the two sides of the tortilla into the center and roll forward to seal.

✳ SUBSTITUTION TIP: In place of the homemade sausage patty, you could use 2 ounces of a good-quality cooked breakfast sausage (preferably turkey).

✳ FLAVOR BOOST: Serve the burrito with a bit of sour cream and Killer Guacamole (page 48). If you like things a little spicier, add a few fresh or pickled jalapeños.

Per serving: Calories: 554; Total Fat: 32g; Saturated Fat: 10g; Protein: 34g; Total Carbohydrates: 34g; Fiber: 6g; Sugar: 3g; Cholesterol: 401mg

BLACK BEAN AND CHORIZO BREAKFAST SKILLET

SERVES: 1   **PREP TIME:** 5 minutes   **COOK TIME:** 35 minutes

You are a man with a big appetite, but sometimes a big meal in the morning makes you feel lazy for the rest of the day. The large portion of roasted sweet potato in this recipe will fill you up without weighing you down, so you can satisfy that hunger and get on with your day.

1 cup diced peeled sweet potato

1 tablespoon olive oil

Salt

Freshly ground black pepper

¼ cup diced Spanish chorizo

¼ cup black bean salsa, homemade (page 49) or store-bought

2 large eggs

2 tablespoons grated cheddar cheese

1. Preheat the oven to 400°F.

2. In a 9-inch ovenproof skillet, combine the sweet potato and olive oil and season with salt and pepper. Toss to combine.

3. Transfer to the oven and roast for 15 minutes. Add the chorizo to the pan and bake for another 10 minutes, or until the sweet potatoes soften.

4. Take the pan out of the oven and spoon the salsa around evenly. Break the eggs into the pan, top with the cheddar, and bake for another 5 to 10 minutes depending on how you like your eggs. Serve hot.

✳ PREP TIP: The sweet potato can be roasted a day ahead or roasted in batches and frozen to cut down on the cooking time of this dish.

Per serving: Calories: 758; Total Fat: 43g; Saturated Fat: 13g; Protein: 28g; Total Carbohydrates: 64g; Fiber: 11g; Sugar: 15g; Cholesterol: 379mg

SAUSAGE AND CHEESE GRITS

SERVES: 2   **PREP TIME:** 5 minutes   **COOK TIME:** 20 minutes

You are a man of true grit. You might as well be eating grits, too. Grits are made of ground corn that has been treated with an alkaline solution to make the corn more digestible. Grits themselves are a staple of Southern cuisine and now you can enjoy them whenever you want.

---

2 tablespoons salted butter, divided

½ cup diced onions

**2 Homemade Turkey Sausage Patties
(page 21)**

½ cup grits or cornmeal

2 cups water

½ cup grated cheddar cheese

Salt

Freshly ground black pepper

---

1. Warm a medium pot over medium-high heat. Add 1 tablespoon of butter and wait until it starts to foam. Add the onions and cook for 3 minutes, or until softened and translucent. Break the sausage patties into small pieces, add to the onions and cook for another 2 minutes to heat the sausage through and develop the flavors.

2. Add the grits and water to the pot. Bring the mixture to a boil, then reduce the heat and cook for 10 to 12 minutes, stirring every minute or so, until the grits are soft.

3. Stir in the cheddar and season with salt and pepper. Serve the grits topped with the remaining 1 tablespoon of butter.

✳ SUBSTITUTION TIP: In place of the homemade sausage patty, you could use 2 ounces of a good-quality cooked breakfast sausage (preferably turkey).

✳ FLAVOR BOOST: For a more substantial meal, top the grits with a poached or fried egg.

Per serving: Calories: 506; Total Fat: 31g; Saturated Fat: 15g; Protein: 23g; Total Carbohydrates: 34g; Fiber: 2g; Sugar: 1g; Cholesterol: 117mg

CLASSIC EGGS BENEDICT

SERVES: 2 **PREP TIME:** 5 minutes **COOK TIME:** 20 minutes

Eggs Benedict is one of those classic dishes that gets blown way out of proportion. So many people think that it's way too difficult to make for them to even try. But you're a smart guy and you're capable. You can wash your own clothes. You can make your own bed. You can do this, too.

---

2 large egg yolks, plus 4 large eggs
½ teaspoon fresh lemon juice
Salt
Freshly ground black pepper
8 tablespoons (1 stick) salted butter, melted
1 teaspoon canola oil
4 slices back bacon
2 English muffins, split in half

---

1. Fill a medium pot with about 3 inches of water. Bring the water to a gentle simmer over medium-low heat.

2. In a medium metal bowl (big enough to sit over the pot of simmering water without falling in), combine the egg yolks, lemon juice, salt, and pepper.

3. Place the bowl over the simmering water and whisk for 3 to 4 minutes, until the yolks start to thicken. Don't stop stirring.

4. Adding only a few drops at a time, whisk the melted butter into the egg yolks until all the butter has been incorporated. Don't add the butter too quickly. Remove the bowl from the heat, whisk for another minute, then cover the bowl with plastic wrap.

5. Break the whole eggs into a small bowl, then gently pour them into the simmering water. Cook the eggs for 6 to 7 minutes, then use a slotted spoon to scoop them out of the water and onto a paper towel.

6. While the eggs are cooking, warm a medium skillet over medium-high heat. Add the oil and cook the bacon for about 2 minutes per side, or until browned on both sides.

7. Toast the English muffins and assemble the eggs Benedict by placing the bacon on the English muffins, putting the eggs on the bacon, and topping with the hollandaise sauce.

FLAVOR BOOST: If you want to class this up even more, you can add some sautéed spinach between the bacon and egg. You can also switch the bacon for smoked salmon. Or you can add 1 tablespoon orange juice to the hollandaise sauce and halve the lemon juice for a touch of sweetness.

Per serving: Calories: 803; Total Fat: 64g; Saturated Fat: 35g; Protein: 31g; Total Carbohydrates: 28g; Fiber: 2g; Sugar: 4g; Cholesterol: 636mg

PEPPERED TOFU SCRAMBLE

SERVES: 2   **PREP TIME:** 5 minutes   **COOK TIME:** 10 minutes

Sometimes you may want to switch things up a little. Maybe you're tired of eggs, or you have a friend over who does not eat eggs. Well, this tofu scramble is the perfect breakfast for those days. Serve the tofu scramble with toast and sliced fruit.

1 tablespoon canola oil

¼ cup diced onion

¼ cup diced green bell pepper

¼ cup diced red bell pepper

Salt

Freshly ground black pepper

1 cup silken tofu

1. Warm a medium nonstick skillet over medium heat. Add the oil, onion, and bell peppers and season with salt and black pepper. Cook the mixture for about 5 minutes, or until the peppers soften and the onions start to turn translucent.

2. Add the tofu, break it up with a spoon, and cook for 3 to 4 more minutes, until the tofu is hot. Serve.

Per serving: Calories: 154; Total Fat: 10g; Saturated Fat: 1g; Protein: 9g; Total Carbohydrates: 7g; Fiber: 1g; Sugar: 4g; Cholesterol: 0mg

GREEN POWER SMOOTHIE

SERVES: 2 **PREP TIME:** 5 minutes

Let's be honest: You wouldn't mind looking a little more Thor-like, right? Well, there's no guarantee that this smoothie will help with that, but there's no guarantee that it won't, either. That sounds like a win-win.

1 cup whole milk

1 cup frozen mango chunks

½ cup packed stemmed spinach

½ cup packed kale leaves (midribs discarded)

½ cup yogurt

In a blender, combine the milk, mango, spinach, kale, and yogurt and puree until it's the consistency of a thick milkshake.

Per serving: Calories: 160; Total Fat: 6g; Saturated Fat: 4g; Protein: 7g; Total Carbohydrates: 20g; Fiber: 1g; Sugar: 19g; Cholesterol: 20mg

BLUE POWER BOOST SMOOTHIE

SERVES: 2   **PREP TIME:** 5 minutes

Feeling a little blue? This smoothie will give you exactly what you need to get up and go. Plus, it tastes really good. What else do you need to know? Right, the recipe . . .

1 cup whole milk

½ cup frozen blueberries

1 banana, cut up

2 tablespoons chia seeds

½ cup yogurt

In a blender, combine the milk, blueberries, banana, chia seeds, and yogurt and puree until it's the consistency of a thick milkshake.

Per serving: Calories: 254; Total Fat: 10g; Saturated Fat: 4g; Protein: 9g; Total Carbohydrates: 34g; Fiber: 8g; Sugar: 21g; Cholesterol: 20mg

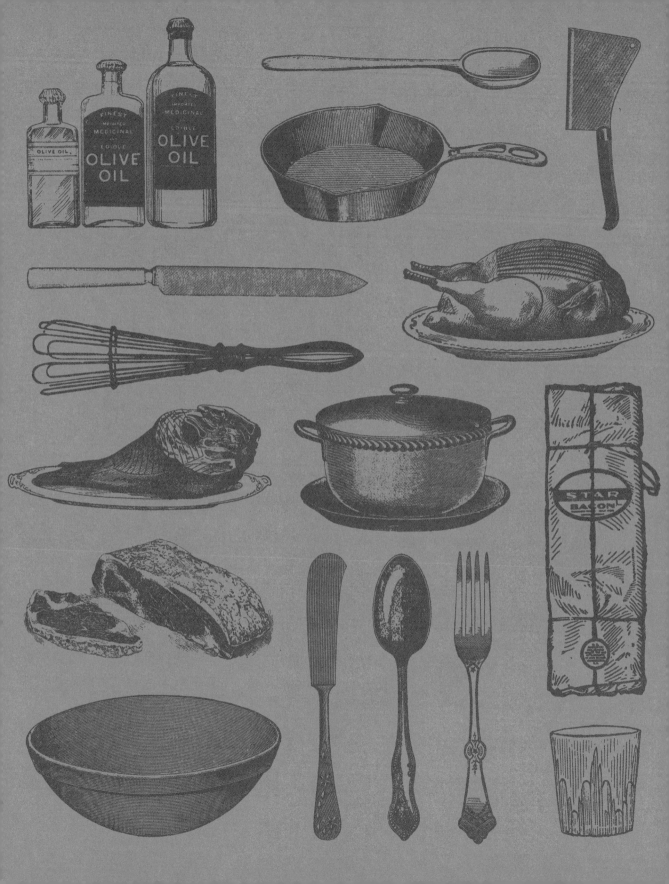

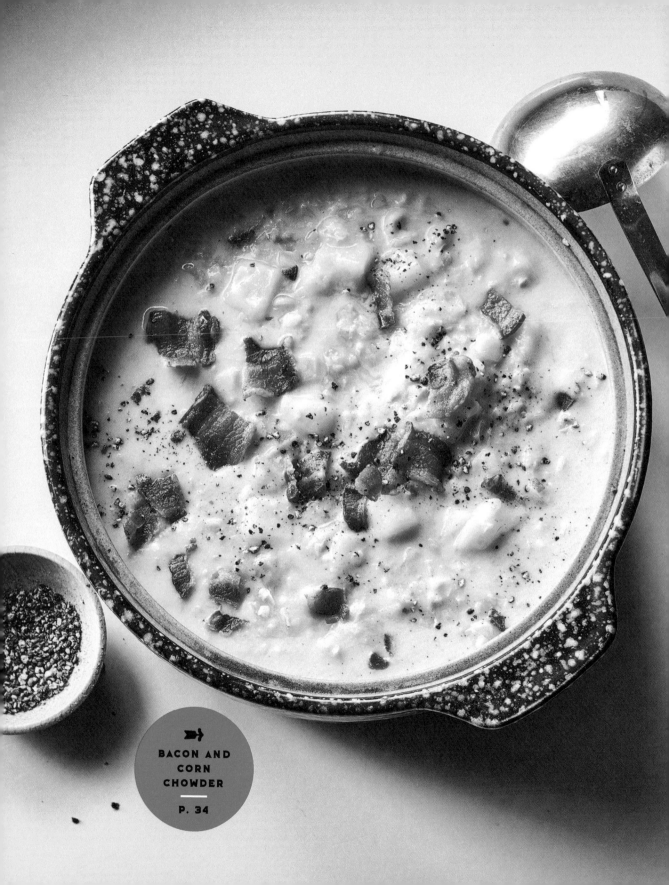

BACON AND
CORN
CHOWDER

P. 34

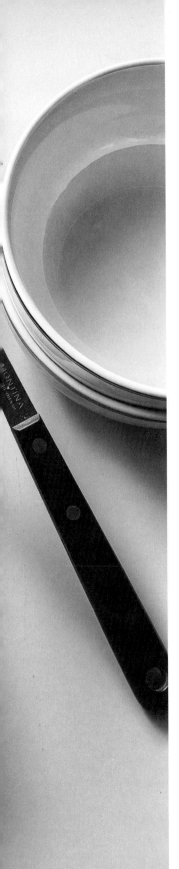

— 3 —

HEARTY SOUPS AND STRONG SALADS

BACON AND CORN CHOWDER

SERVES: 4 **PREP TIME:** 10 minutes **COOK TIME:** 35 minutes

This corn chowder is the ultimate comfort food. It comes together quickly, it will fill you up, and it tastes delicious. This is the thing to turn to on a cold winter day, or after a hard day at the office.

1 cup diced peeled potatoes
Salt
4 slices bacon, diced
1 baseball-size onion, diced
1 (14-ounce) can cream-style corn
3 cups whole milk
Freshly ground black pepper

1. Put the potatoes in a medium pot and add water to cover them by 2 inches. Season the water with salt, bring it to a boil over high heat, and cook the potatoes for about 12 minutes, or until they are soft. Drain the potatoes and set them aside.

2. Rinse out the pot and put it back on the stove over medium heat. Add the bacon to the pot and cook for 5 minutes. Add the onion to the bacon and cook for another 5 minutes.

3. Carefully drain off the bacon fat, leaving the bacon in the pan. Add the cream-style corn and milk to the pot and heat the chowder over medium heat for about 10 minutes, or until it's hot. Do not boil! Add the cooked potatoes to the chowder and let them cook for 2 minutes to absorb some of the flavor. Season the chowder with salt and pepper and serve.

Per serving: Calories: 270; Total Fat: 9g; Saturated Fat: 5g; Protein: 12g; Total Carbohydrates: 39g; Fiber: 2g; Sugar: 14g; Cholesterol: 26mg

CHICKEN NOODLE SOUP

SERVES: 4 **PREP TIME:** 10 minutes **COOK TIME:** 45 minutes

Feeling sick? Chicken noodle soup. Feeling sad? Chicken noodle soup. Aliens are taking over the planet and you must convince a ragtag group of outcasts to come together for the good of all humans? Chicken noodle soup. For every problem, chicken noodle soup.

---

4 ounces pad thai–style rice noodles

2 whole bone-in chicken legs (drumstick and thigh)

8 cups water

1 teaspoon salt, plus more to taste

1 tablespoon olive oil

1 cup thinly sliced onion

½ cup sliced celery

½ cup sliced carrots

Freshly ground black pepper

Per serving: Calories: 224; Total Fat: 6g; Saturated Fat: 1g; Protein: 13g; Total Carbohydrates: 29g; Fiber: 2g; Sugar: 3g; Cholesterol: 50mg

1. Cook the rice noodles according to the package directions, then run under cold water to cool.

2. Put the chicken legs in a medium pot. Add the water and 1 teaspoon salt, and bring to a boil. Reduce the heat to low and simmer for 20 minutes.

3. Set a large sieve over a large heatproof bowl. Pour the liquid and chicken into the sieve. Set aside the chicken and the cooking liquid. When the chicken is cool enough to handle, pull the meat off the bones and pull it into shreds. Discard the skin and bones.

4. Return the pot to medium-high heat. Add the oil, onion, celery, and carrots and cook for 7 to 8 minutes, until the vegetables are softened. Add the chicken cooking liquid to the pot and bring to a boil. Reduce the heat to a simmer and cook for 10 minutes.

5. Taste the soup and season with salt and pepper until it tastes good. Divide the noodles among 4 bowls and top with the pulled chicken. Ladle the soup over the bowls of noodles and go save the world from those pesky aliens, you hero.

FIRE-ROASTED TOMATO SOUP

SERVES: 4   **PREP TIME:** 20 minutes   **COOK TIME:** 45 minutes

There are few things better in this world than fire-roasted tomato soup and a grilled cheese. It is no 20-year-old Pappy Reserve, but it's pretty good. Serve the soup with The Ultimate Grilled Cheese (page 55).

---

6 Roma (plum) tomatoes

3 tablespoons olive oil, divided

1 cup diced onion

2 tablespoons minced garlic (about 2 large cloves)

4 cups whole milk

¼ cup thinly sliced fresh basil

Salt

Freshly ground black pepper

✳ **PREP TIP:** If you don't have a grill, you can roast the tomatoes in the oven. Preheat the oven to 400°F. Halve the tomatoes lengthwise, drizzle them with olive oil, and place them cut-side up on a parchment-lined sheet pan. Bake them, without flipping over, for 30 to 35 minutes. Transfer to a bowl, cover, and peel as directed above.

1. Heat the grill to 450°F.

2. Drizzle the whole tomatoes with 1 tablespoon of olive oil and throw them on the grill. Cook the tomatoes for 12 to 15 minutes, turning every 2 minutes, until charred around the edges and soft in the middle.

3. Put the roasted tomatoes in a large bowl and cover very tightly with plastic wrap. Let the tomatoes sit for 10 minutes, then peel off and discard the skin.

4. Warm a large pot over medium-high heat. Add 2 tablespoons of olive oil and the onion and sauté for 5 minutes, or until softened. Add the garlic and cook for another minute.

5. Add the tomatoes and milk, reduce the heat to medium-low, and simmer for 20 minutes (do not boil!).

6. Remove from the heat, add the basil, and blast the whole thing with an immersion blender. (Or do this in a regular blender, but take the steam vent out of the center of the lid and cover the hole with a towel.)

7. Taste the soup and season with salt and pepper until it tastes good. Serve hot.

Per serving: Calories: 275; Total Fat: 18g; Saturated Fat: 6g; Protein: 9g; Total Carbohydrates: 20g; Fiber: 2g; Sugar: 17g; Cholesterol: 24mg

MANLY TOMATO VEGETABLE SOUP

SERVES: 6 **PREP TIME:** 10 minutes **COOK TIME:** 30 minutes

This soup is simple and quick to throw together. It's also loaded with vegetables, because not every meal can be steak. You can feel good about eating it because it's good for you. It also happens to taste great and will leave you feeling full and satisfied.

1 tablespoon olive oil

2 cups diced onion

1 cup diced celery

1 (14.5-ounce) can crushed tomatoes

2 cups diced white potatoes

1 cup frozen vegetable medley (carrot, peas, corn)

12 cups water

Salt

Freshly ground black pepper

1. Warm a large pot over medium-high heat. Add the oil, onion, and celery and cook for 5 minutes. Throw in the tomatoes, potatoes, frozen vegetables, and water. Bring to a boil, then reduce the heat to low and simmer for 20 minutes, or until the potatoes are tender.

2. Taste the soup and season it with salt and pepper as you see fit.

✳ FLAVOR BOOST: As a man, you're building muscles every day. It could be your arm muscles, your back muscles, or your brain muscles. To help build those muscles, you may want a little extra protein. Hit this soup with a 15-ounce can of chickpeas and watch those muscles grow.

Per serving: Calories: 119; Total Fat: 3g; Saturated Fat: 1g; Protein: 4g; Total Carbohydrates: 22g; Fiber: 4g; Sugar: 8g; Cholesterol: 0mg

WHITE BEAN AND CHORIZO SOUP

SERVES: 6 **PREP TIME:** 10 minutes **COOK TIME:** 45 minutes

Chorizo is a Spanish-style sausage flavored heavily with paprika. That heavy paprika taste is the key to flavoring a big a pot of soup with only a handful of ingredients. Not only does this soup have a bold taste, but the beans and sausage provide a big hit of protein and make for a filling meal.

1 tablespoon olive oil

1 cup diced onion

1 cup diced celery

2 garlic cloves, sliced

1 cup diced Spanish chorizo

1 (15.5-ounce) can cannellini beans, drained and rinsed

12 cups water

Salt

Freshly ground black pepper

1. Warm a large pot over medium-high heat. Add the oil, onion, celery, garlic, and chorizo and cook for 10 minutes, or until the vegetables are tender and lightly browned.

2. Add the beans, water, and salt and pepper to taste. Bring to a boil, then reduce the heat to low and simmer the soup for 30 minutes.

3. Taste the soup, season with more salt and pepper if needed, and serve.

Per serving: Calories: 209; Total Fat: 13g; Saturated Fat: 4g; Protein: 9g; Total Carbohydrates: 15g; Fiber: 4g; Sugar: 3g; Cholesterol: 24mg

HOT AND SOUR SOUP

SERVES: 6 **PREP TIME:** 10 minutes, plus 30 minutes to soak **COOK TIME:** 30 minutes

This Sichuan-esque hot and sour soup is not strictly authentic. The real version would be seasoned with vinegar and pepper. In this version, to cut down on ingredients, we'll use the chile paste called sambal oelek, because it is both acidic and spicy.

½ cup dried shiitake mushrooms

12 cups water, divided

1 tablespoon olive oil

1 pound ground pork

1 cup diced onion

2 tablespoons sambal oelek

2 tablespoons soy sauce

Salt

Freshly ground black pepper

1. Soak the shiitake mushrooms in 4 cups of water in a medium bowl for 30 minutes.

2. Warm a large pot over medium-high heat. Add the olive oil, pork, and onion. Cook for 7 to 8 minutes, until the pork is browned and the onions are translucent.

3. Scoop the mushrooms out of the water and slice them nice and thin. Pour the mushroom soaking water, plus the remaining 8 cups of water into the pot. Add the mushrooms along with the sambal, soy sauce, and salt and pepper to taste.

4. Bring the soup to a boil, then reduce the heat to low and simmer for 20 minutes to develop the flavors. Serve.

✳ FLAVOR BOOST: In true hot and sour soup fashion, you can gently stir 2 beaten eggs into this soup a few minutes before serving to create egg "noodles."

✳ SUBSTITUTION TIP: If you can't find dried shiitakes, substitute another dried mushroom rather than fresh ones. Fresh mushrooms will not give this soup the same concentrated flavors as the dried ones do.

Per serving: Calories: 209; Total Fat: 14g; Saturated Fat: 4g; Protein: 15g; Total Carbohydrates: 5g; Fiber: 2g; Sugar: 2g; Cholesterol: 51mg

HAMBURGER SOUP

SERVES: 4   **PREP TIME:** 5 minutes   **COOK TIME:** 30 minutes

Making hamburger soup is a great way to use leftover hamburgers from the previous day's barbecue. Because the burgers are grilled, the soup takes on a slightly smoky flavor that you won't get from using fresh ground beef.

1 tablespoon olive oil

½ cup diced onion

1 (14.5-ounce) can crushed tomatoes

8 cups beef stock

1 cup (½-inch) diced white potato

2 cooked burger patties (The Burger, page 59)

Salt

Freshly ground black pepper

1. Warm a large pot over medium-high heat. Add the oil and onion and cook for 8 minutes, or until the onion starts to brown.

2. Add the tomatoes, beef stock, and potatoes. Bring to a boil and cook for 10 minutes.

3. Break the burgers into bite-size pieces and throw them into the soup. Reduce the heat to low and simmer for 10 more minutes.

4. Taste the soup and season with salt and pepper until you think it tastes good.

FLAVOR BOOST: Add a 15-ounce can of white beans to the soup to make it a little more substantial. Additionally, you can top the soup with a few tablespoons of grated cheddar cheese, because why wouldn't you?

Per serving: Calories: 249; Total Fat: 13g; Saturated Fat: 4g; Protein: 17g; Total Carbohydrates: 16g; Fiber: 3g; Sugar: 6g; Cholesterol: 34mg

ROASTED VEGETABLE AND GOAT CHEESE SALAD

SERVES: 2   **PREP TIME:** 15 minutes

There's something magical about the combination of balsamic vinegar, roasted vegetables, and goat cheese. Consider this salad a rabbit in your hat that you can pull out when you need it because it is utterly amazing.

Roasted Vegetables (page 90)
2 tablespoons balsamic vinegar
2 cups baby arugula
¼ cup crumbled goat cheese
1 tablespoon olive oil
Salt
Freshly ground black pepper

---

1. Put the roasted vegetables in a medium bowl. Add the balsamic and toss to coat. Let the vegetables marinate for 10 minutes.

2. Add the arugula to the bowl and stir using a set of tongs. Plate the salad, top with the goat cheese, drizzle with the olive oil, and season with salt and pepper.

Per serving: Calories: 474; Total Fat: 34g; Saturated Fat: 12g; Protein: 14g; Total Carbohydrates: 29g; Fiber: 5g; Sugar: 13g; Cholesterol: 36mg

SOUTHWEST SALAD

SERVES: 1 **PREP TIME:** 5 minutes

What is there to say about a salad that's so simple and so delicious? I guess that's it: This salad is simple and delicious. You're going to love it even though it's a salad.

2 cups bite-size pieces iceberg lettuce

¼ cup canned or frozen corn kernels, cooked

2 tablespoons Creamy Avocado-Lime Dressing (page 146)

¼ cup black bean salsa, homemade (page 49) or store-bought

2 tablespoons grated cheddar cheese

In a medium bowl, combine the lettuce, corn, and dressing. Stir using a set of tongs to coat the lettuce. Put the salad in a serving bowl and top with the black bean salsa and cheddar.

SUBSTITUTION TIP: Although the avocado-lime dressing is highly recommended, you could make this salad with a store-bought ranch dressing.

FLAVOR BOOST: Roast pork, chicken, or beef as well as bell peppers, poblano peppers, cherry tomatoes, or rice can be added to this salad to make it more of a meal.

Per serving: Calories: 218; Total Fat: 13g; Saturated Fat: 4g; Protein: 7g; Total Carbohydrates: 19g; Fiber: 5g; Sugar: 6g; Cholesterol: 18mg

CLASSIC-ISH NIÇOISE SALAD

SERVES: 2 **PREP TIME:** 10 minutes **COOK TIME:** 5 minutes

A classic Niçoise salad is typically a combination of green beans, olives, tomatoes, tuna, potatoes, and boiled eggs. This version is simplified by taking away the potatoes and eggs and removing all of the cooking except the green beans.

1 pound green beans

¼ cup water

1 cup cherry tomatoes, halved

½ cup Niçoise olives

¼ cup Basic Vinaigrette (page 147) or
   store-bought Italian dressing

1 (5-ounce) can tuna, drained

Salt

Freshly ground black pepper

1. Put the green beans and water in a microwave-safe container and cover tightly with plastic wrap. Microwave on high for 2 minutes. Poke a hole in the plastic wrap with a knife to release the steam, then remove the wrap, drain the water off the beans, and rinse them under cold water for 2 minutes.

2. Put the green beans in a medium bowl along with the tomatoes, olives, and vinaigrette. Toss to coat.

3. Add the tuna and gently stir into the salad. Season with salt and pepper and serve.

✳ FLAVOR BOOST: To make the salad more substantial, add 1 cup spinach, and 1 cup cooked penne noodles.

Per serving: Calories: 380; Total Fat: 24g; Saturated Fat: 4g; Protein: 22g; Total Carbohydrates: 24g; Fiber: 8g; Sugar: 11g; Cholesterol: 19mg

SOBA NOODLE SALAD

SERVES: 2 **PREP TIME:** 10 minutes

Soba are traditional Japanese buckwheat noodles that are often served cold in the summer and hot in the winter. They are a chewy, hearty noodle that make a perfect base for a salad.

2 cups cooked soba noodles (follow the package directions), rinsed in cold water

½ cup grated carrot

½ cup thinly sliced bok choy

½ cup thinly sliced red bell pepper

¼ cup sesame-ginger dressing, homemade (page 148) or store-bought

In a medium bowl, toss together the noodles, carrot, bok choy, and bell pepper. Add the dressing and toss to coat the noodles and vegetables.

SUBSTITUTION TIP: If you can't find bok choy at the grocery store, you can substitute it with any kind of cabbage, as long as it's very thinly sliced.

FLAVOR BOOST: To add a little color to the final salad, garnish it with black and white sesame seeds and thinly sliced scallions.

Per serving: Calories: 314; Total Fat: 10g; Saturated Fat: 1g; Protein: 9g; Total Carbohydrates: 52g; Fiber: 2g; Sugar: 7g; Cholesterol: 0mg

ARUGULA AND PROSCIUTTO SALAD

SERVES: 2 **PREP TIME:** 5 minutes

What's the point of learning to cook if you can't show off once in a while? This is the salad that you do that with. It's super simple, exceptionally delicious, and it looks like something from a five-star restaurant.

2 cups baby arugula

1 green apple, thinly sliced

3 tablespoons Basic Vinaigrette (page 147) or store-bought Italian dressing

2 slices prosciutto

Salt

Freshly ground black pepper

¼ cup shaved Parmesan cheese

1. In a medium bowl, toss the arugula and apple with the dressing.

2. Divide the salad between two plates. Gently scrunch up the prosciutto slices and place one on each plate beside the salad.

3. Season the salad with salt and pepper and finish it with the Parmesan shavings.

※ INGREDIENT TIP: Buy a chunk of Parmesan cheese rather than the grated stuff. It will have more flavor and you will get more bang for your buck. Don't worry about it going bad—it will last in your fridge for months. Use a vegetable peeler to make the Parmesan shavings (which also make a fantastic garnish for a bowl of pasta).

Per serving: Calories: 251; Total Fat: 18g; Saturated Fat: 4g; Protein: 7g; Total Carbohydrates: 17g; Fiber: 3g; Sugar: 12g; Cholesterol: 16mg

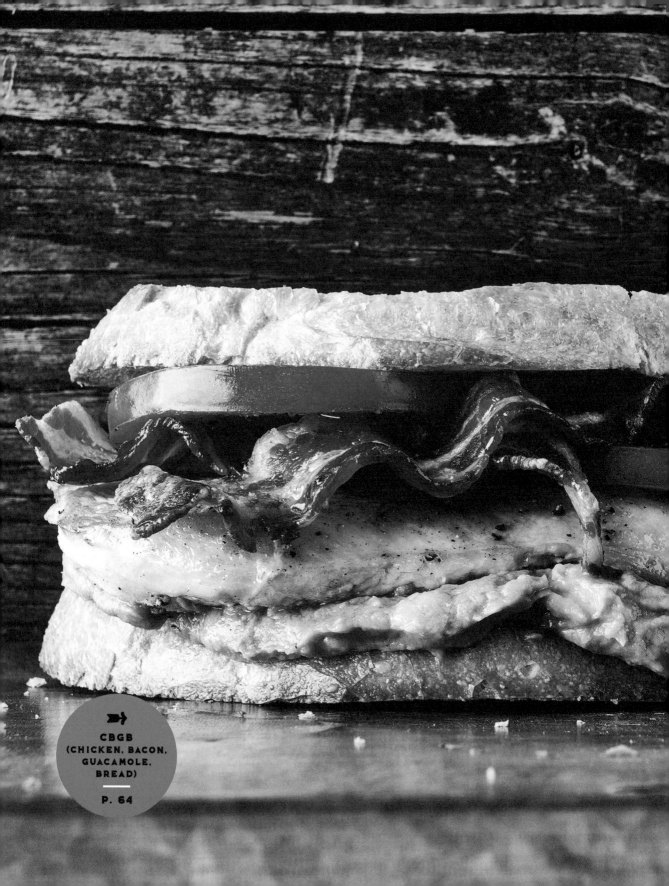

CBGB
(CHICKEN, BACON,
GUACAMOLE,
BREAD)

P. 64

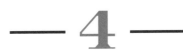

STUDLY SNACKS, WRAPS, AND SANDWICHES

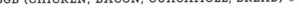

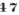

KILLER GUACAMOLE

MAKES: 1½ cups   **PREP TIME:** 10 minutes

Guacamole is obviously fantastic to eat with nachos and tacos, but it's also a great on wraps, sandwiches, and burgers. You can never go wrong mixing a batch and throwing it in the fridge.

1 cup diced avocado (about 2 avocados)
Juice of 1 lime, plus more to taste
2 tablespoons minced red onion
2 tablespoons diced tomato
1 tablespoon chopped fresh cilantro
¼ teaspoon salt, plus more to taste

In a medium bowl, combine the avocado, lime juice, red onion, tomato, cilantro, and salt and mash it all together using a potato masher until it's smooth. Taste the guacamole and add a little more lime juice and salt to suit your taste.

✳ STORAGE TIP: Store the guacamole in a plastic or ceramic container with a layer of plastic wrap pressed flat against the surface of the guacamole. Cover the container tightly with a second piece of plastic wrap. This will help prevent browning on the surface.

Per serving (½ cup): Calories: 75; Total Fat: 6g; Saturated Fat: 1g; Protein: 1g; Total Carbohydrates: 6g; Fiber: 3g; Sugar: 1g; Cholesterol: 0mg

BALLIN' BLACK BEAN SALSA

MAKES: 4 cups **PREP TIME:** 10 minutes, plus overnight to cool
COOK TIME: 30 minutes

This black bean salsa has a kick that you can't resist. You can scoop it up with chips, throw it in a breakfast skillet, or use it to top a tasty taco. This is the perfect thing for when your friends are over to watch the big game.

2 teaspoons olive oil

1 baseball-size onion, diced

1 (12-ounce) can pickled jalapeños, drained

1 (15-ounce) can black beans, drained and rinsed

1 (14.5-ounce) can diced tomatoes, drained

2 tablespoons chopped cilantro

Salt

Freshly ground black pepper

1. In a medium pot, warm the olive oil over medium heat. Add the onion and cook for 5 minutes, or until translucent. Add the jalapeños and cook for 2 more minutes.

2. Throw in the black beans and tomatoes and bring to a boil. Reduce the heat to low and simmer the salsa for 15 to 20 minutes, or until thick.

3. Remove from the heat and stir in the cilantro. Taste and season with salt and pepper. Put the salsa in a container and cool in the fridge overnight.

Per serving (½ cup): Calories: 88; Total Fat: 1g; Saturated Fat: <1g; Protein: 4g; Total Carbohydrates: 14g; Fiber: 5g; Sugar: 2g; Cholesterol: 0mg

HUNGRY, HUNGRY HUMMUS

    (30) (DF) (x2) (GF) (OP) (VG)

MAKES: 2 cups   **PREP TIME:** 10 minutes

Bro, are you still buying hummus? Seriously? Here's a little secret: Hummus is super easy to make. The homemade stuff is way better than the store-bought stuff and it's also way cheaper. Really, it's a no-brainer.

1 (15.5-ounce) can chickpeas, drained and rinsed

2 teaspoons minced garlic

1 tablespoon fresh lemon juice, plus more to taste

¼ teaspoon ground cumin

1 tablespoon tahini

1 tablespoon olive oil

¼ teaspoon salt, plus more to taste

2 to 3 tablespoons water

In a food processor, combine the chickpeas, garlic, lemon juice, cumin, tahini, olive oil, and salt. Pulse for about 30 seconds. Run the food processor on high and slowly pour in enough water to make the hummus smooth and creamy. Taste the hummus, and, if it needs it, hit it with a bit more salt and lemon juice.

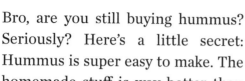 **SUBSTITUTION TIP:** Tahini is like peanut butter but made with sesame seeds. If you cannot find tahini, don't worry. You can sub in another kind of nut butter, such as peanut, almond, or cashew.

Per serving (½ cup): Calories: 178; Total Fat: 11g; Saturated Fat: 1g; Protein: 5g; Total Carbohydrates: 16g; Fiber: 5g; Sugar: 3g; Cholesterol: 0mg

SPICED NUTS

MAKES: 2 cups   **PREP TIME:** 5 minutes, plus 1 hour to cool   **COOK TIME:** 10 minutes

Spiced nuts not only make a great snack, but they're also awesome to throw on a salad. They last a long time—as long as they are in an airtight container—so you can double, triple, quadruple, or whatever five times this recipe is. Either way, you're gonna love these nuts.

¾ cup sugar, divided

1 teaspoon garam masala

¼ teaspoon salt

2 cups unsalted mixed nuts

½ cup water

1. In a medium bowl, combine ¼ cup of sugar, the garam masala, and salt. Set aside.

2. Warm a medium skillet over medium-high heat. Add the nuts and roast them, keeping them moving, for about 4 minutes, or until they start to brown.

3. Pour the remaining ½ cup of sugar over the nuts along with the water. Bring the mixture to a boil, reduce the heat to medium, and cook until the mixture starts to turn a light brown, usually within 3 minutes.

4. Use a slotted spoon to take the nuts out of the pan and put them in the bowl with the sugar and spice. Toss the nuts to evenly coat them.

5. Spread the nuts out on a baking sheet and let cool for 1 hour. Store the nuts in an airtight container.

✱ **INGREDIENT TIP:** Garam masala is a common Indian spice blend made of cinnamon, clove, star anise, cardamom, and a few other ingredients. You can generally find it in the spice aisle at your local grocery store, but for the really good stuff head to a specialty Indian market.

Per serving (½ cup): Calories: 589; Total Fat: 41g; Saturated Fat: 7g; Protein: 11g; Total Carbohydrates: 54g; Fiber: 4g; Sugar: 41g; Cholesterol: 0mg

BACON AND BLUE CROSTINI

MAKES: 12 crostini   **PREP TIME:** 10 minutes   **COOK TIME:** 30 minutes

Bacon, good. Blue cheese, good. When you add pear to the mix, things somehow get even better. And, when you spread it all on a toasted baguette you might as well be David Copperfield because you just made magic, my man. Let's do this.

---

12 slices (¼ inch thick) baguette

2 tablespoons olive oil

Salt

Freshly ground black pepper

4 slices bacon, diced

2 Bosc pears, peeled and diced

2 tablespoons water

1 tablespoon sugar

½ cup crumbled blue cheese, at room temperature

---

1. Preheat the oven to 350°F.

2. Arrange the baguette slices on a sheet pan and drizzle them with the olive oil. Season the bread with salt and pepper and bake for 10 to 12 minutes, until the bread is crisp.

3. Warm a medium skillet over medium heat and add the bacon. Cook for about 5 minutes.

4. Drain off all but 1 tablespoon of the bacon fat. Add the pears to the pan and cook for 2 minutes. Add the water and sugar and cook for 8 to 10 minutes, until the mixture is thick. Remove from the heat and let cool.

5. Spread a thin layer of blue cheese on each of the crostini. Top the cheese with the cooled bacon and pear mixture. Say "Voilà!" and enjoy.

Per serving (1 crostini): Calories: 168; Total Fat: 6g; Saturated Fat: 3g; Protein: 6g; Total Carbohydrates: 22g; Fiber: 1g; Sugar: 4g; Cholesterol: 10mg

FIRE-ROASTED RED PEPPER DIP

MAKES: 2 cups   **PREP TIME:** 35 minutes, plus time to cool   **COOK TIME:** 15 minutes

This is a classic Greek dip with a twist. The addition of mint and jalapeño adds a kick of flavor that will leave you wanting more for weeks after you've eaten it. This is a little salty, a little sweet, a little spicy, and a lot delicious. For this recipe the peppers can be roasted in the oven on 400°F for about 35 minutes rather than on the grill. Serve the dip with grilled pita bread.

2 red bell peppers

1 jalapeño pepper

1 cup crumbled feta cheese

1 tablespoon chopped fresh mint

1 to 2 tablespoons olive oil

Salt

Freshly ground black pepper

1. Heat the grill to high. Put the red bell peppers and jalapeño on the grill and roast for about 15 minutes, turning every 2 to 3 minutes, until the skin of the peppers is completely black.

2. Put the peppers in a metal bowl and cover very tightly with plastic wrap. Let sit for 10 minutes.

3. Rub the peppers with a kitchen towel to remove the skins. Remove the stems and seeds from the peppers and discard. Let the peppers cool to room temperature.

4. Transfer the peppers to a food processor and add the feta, mint, and 1 tablespoon of olive oil. Pulse the mixture until it is completely combined. Add the remaining 1 tablespoon of oil if the mixture isn't coming together. Season with salt and black pepper to taste.

✱ SUBSTITUTION TIP: Instead of roasting your own peppers, you can buy them jarred at the grocery store. This will save you on time and cleanup. Just make sure to drain the store-bought peppers very well because the liquid they come packed in will thin out the dip.

Per serving (½ cup): Calories: 176; Total Fat: 15g; Saturated Fat: 6g; Protein: 6g; Total Carbohydrates: 5g; Fiber: 1g; Sugar: 4g; Cholesterol: 33mg

BROCCOLI SNACKERS

SERVES: 2   **PREP TIME:** 5 minutes   **COOK TIME:** 20 minutes

What do you get when you take broccoli, toss it with olive oil, hit it with Parmesan cheese and red pepper flakes, roast it, then finish it with lemon juice? You get a delicious and healthy snack that you won't be able to stop eating. With these broccoli snackers, you'll get your full daily dose of vegetables in the best way possible.

2 cups broccoli florets

1 tablespoon olive oil

¼ cup grated Parmesan cheese

¼ teaspoon red pepper flakes

¼ teaspoon salt

2 teaspoons fresh lemon juice

1. Preheat the oven to 400°F. Line a sheet pan with parchment paper or aluminum foil.

2. In a medium bowl, combine the broccoli, olive oil, Parmesan, pepper flakes, and salt. Toss to evenly coat the broccoli.

3. Spread the broccoli on the lined pan and roast for 17 to 20 minutes, until the broccoli is slightly dark and crisp.

4. Squeeze the lemon juice over the broccoli and eat.

✳ PREP TIP: To make prepping easier and a lot less messy, cut the broccoli into florets through the stem ends rather than through the floret tops.

Per serving: Calories: 139; Total Fat: 10g; Saturated Fat: 3g; Protein: 6g; Total Carbohydrates: 6g; Fiber: 2g; Sugar: 1g; Cholesterol: 11mg

THE ULTIMATE GRILLED CHEESE

SERVES: 2 **PREP TIME:** 5 minutes **COOK TIME:** 10 minutes

A good grilled cheese is a thing of beauty. The gooey, melty cheese, the crispy golden-brown bread. It brings a tear to the eye. Oh, nope, it's just a stray drop of whiskey. Anyway, this is good, like *really* good.

---

5 tablespoons salted butter, at room temperature, divided

4 slices sourdough bread

2 slices applewood smoked cheddar cheese

2 slices Swiss cheese

2 slices provolone cheese

---

1. Butter each of the 4 slices of bread on one side with 1 tablespoon of butter.

2. Heat a large skillet over medium heat. Add the remaining 1 tablespoon of butter to the pan and throw 2 slices of bread in, butter-side up. Cook the bread for 1 minute.

3. Flip the bread butter-side down and top each with a slice of cheddar, Swiss, and provolone cheese. Top with the remaining bread, butter-side up. Cook the sandwich on one side until the bread is golden brown, then flip and do the same thing on the other side.

4. Take the grilled cheeses out of the pan and put them on a wire rack to chill out for 2 minutes, then cut and serve.

Per serving: Calories: 735; Total Fat: 50g; Saturated Fat: 31g; Protein: 26g; Total Carbohydrates: 45g; Fiber: 2g; Sugar: 4g; Cholesterol: 135mg

HEFTY VEGGIE WRAP

    (VG)

SERVES: 1 **PREP TIME:** 5 minutes

Just because you want to eat vegetables sometimes doesn't mean you don't also want to feel full. This wrap will fill up your veggie quota and your belly, so you have the energy to do what you want.

2 tablespoons hummus, homemade (page 50) or store-bought
1 (12-inch) whole wheat tortilla
1 cup Roasted Vegetables (page 90)
1 cup baby spinach

Spread the hummus evenly on the tortilla. Put the vegetables in the center of the tortilla and top with the spinach. Roll the bottom of the tortilla up over the vegetables, then fold the sides into the center. Pull back on the rolled tortilla to tighten it, then roll forward to finish the wrap.

❋ SUBSTITUTION TIP: The roasted vegetables can be substituted with jarred roasted red pepper and canned artichoke hearts.

Per serving: Calories: 505; Total Fat: 20g; Saturated Fat: 5g; Protein: 11g; Total Carbohydrates: 75g; Fiber: 7g; Sugar: 12g; Cholesterol: 0mg

SWEET POTATO TACOS

SERVES: 1 **PREP TIME:** 10 minutes **COOK TIME:** 25 minutes

Tacos without meat? You've got to be kidding! Nope, and you're going to love them. It may help if you think of these, not as tacos, but as open-faced quesadillas. Just eat them—you'll like them.

---

1 small sweet potato (the size of a pair of balled-up socks)

1 teaspoon salt

3 (4-inch) corn tortillas

¼ cup grated Monterey Jack cheese

¼ cup black bean salsa, homemade (page 49) or store-bought

2 tablespoons sour cream

---

1. Put the sweet potato in a medium pot, and add cold water to cover by at least 1 inch. Add the salt, bring to a boil, and cook the sweet potato for about 20 minutes, or until a knife slides easily through the center of it.

2. Drain the sweet potato and let it cool until you can handle it with your bare hands. Peel it and slice it into finger-size pieces.

3. Warm a nonstick skillet over medium heat. Put the tortillas in the pan and heat for 45 seconds. Flip the tortillas and top with the cheese. Once the cheese starts to melt, flip the tortillas and cook for another minute, or until the cheese is browned.

4. Remove the cheesy tortillas from the pan and top the cheesy side with sweet potato, black bean salsa, and sour cream.

✳ FLAVOR BOOST: If you really want to turn these tacos up to 11, add some guacamole, fresh cilantro, and jalapeño. Hell, why not add a squeeze of fresh lime juice while you're at it? That's how you turn good into great.

Per serving: Calories: 418; Total Fat: 16g; Saturated Fat: 8g; Protein: 14g; Total Carbohydrates: 54g; Fiber: 9g; Sugar: 10g; Cholesterol: 42mg

RIB EYE TACOS

SERVES: 1 **PREP TIME:** 5 minutes, plus 5 minutes to rest **COOK TIME:** 10 minutes

There's a good chance that you get the craving for steak every once in a while (unless you're vegetarian, of course). Well, what better way to eat steak than wrapped in a tortilla with onion, cilantro, and jalapeño? There is no better way—that's the answer.

1 teaspoon olive oil

1 (5-ounce) rib eye steak

Salt

Freshly ground black pepper

3 (4-inch) corn tortillas

2 tablespoons minced white onion

1 tablespoon chopped fresh cilantro

1 jalapeño pepper, thinly sliced

1. Warm a heavy skillet over medium-high heat. Add the olive oil. Season the steak well with salt and pepper and cook for 4 minutes per side. Remove the steak from the pan and let it rest for 5 minutes.

2. Heat the tortillas in the steak pan for 30 seconds per side.

3. Slice the steak thin and divide among the tortillas. Top the steak with onion, cilantro, and jalapeño.

FLAVOR BOOST: Serve the tacos with your favorite Mexican hot sauce and sour cream.

Per serving: Calories: 506; Total Fat: 31g; Saturated Fat: 11g; Protein: 30g; Total Carbohydrates: 22g; Fiber: 4g; Sugar: 3g; Cholesterol: 95mg

THE BURGER

SERVES: 4 **PREP TIME:** 10 minutes **COOK TIME:** 10 minutes

This is simply called The Burger because it's the only burger you'll ever need. This recipe is the best base burger recipe. It has loads of flavor and will make the perfect platform for whatever crazy toppings you want to throw on top of it.

1 pound ground beef (80% lean)

½ teaspoon garlic powder

½ teaspoon onion powder

¼ teaspoon salt

¼ teaspoon freshly ground black pepper

4 burger buns

1. In a medium bowl, combine the ground beef, garlic powder, onion powder, salt, and pepper. Wet your hands with cold water and mix to combine.

2. Wet your hands with cold water again, divide the meat into 4 portions, and roll into balls. Form the balls into patties about ¼ inch thick.

3. Heat the grill to 400°F for 15 minutes. Grill the patties for 3 to 4 minutes per side.

4. Toast the buns, put a burger on each, top with your favorite condiments, and enjoy.

❋ **PREP TIP:** You can also cook the burgers in a skillet over medium-high heat for 4 to 5 minutes per side.

Per serving: Calories: 418; Total Fat: 21g; Saturated Fat: 8g; Protein: 27g; Total Carbohydrates: 29g; Fiber: 1g; Sugar: 4g; Cholesterol: 68mg

THE COWBOY BURGER

SERVES: 2 **PREP TIME:** 10 minutes **COOK TIME:** 10 minutes

This is a big burger for a big appetite. It's two patties, cheese, onions, and horseradish mayo. Historical records show that this is the exact burger cowboys used to eat in the Wild West. Okay, that might not be true, but it's what an old-timey cowboy would eat if they were here right now.

---

1 tablespoon prepared horseradish

¼ cup mayonnaise

1 tablespoon olive oil

1 softball-size onion, thinly sliced

¼ teaspoon salt

2 burger buns

4 cooked burger patties (The Burger, page 59)

---

1. In a small bowl, stir together the horseradish and mayonnaise. Set aside.

2. Heat a medium skillet over medium-high heat. Add the olive oil, onion, and salt to the pan and cook for 10 minutes, or until the onions are softened and browned.

3. Toast the buns in the pan and spread the top and bottom halves of each bun with the horseradish mayo. Put a cooked patty on each of the bottom buns, and top each with a quarter of the onions. Set a second patty on top of the onions and top with the remaining onions. Add the top bun.

✳ **INGREDIENT TIP:** Prepared horseradish is the stuff you buy in the little bottle at the grocery store. The horseradish is cooked with vinegar and a few other ingredients to add a touch of acidity and to mellow out some of the spiciness.

Per serving: Calories: 949; Total Fat: 66g; Saturated Fat: 20g; Protein: 50g; Total Carbohydrates: 36g; Fiber: 2g; Sugar: 7g; Cholesterol: 148mg

THE KICKIN' CHICKEN SANDWICH

SERVES: 1 **PREP TIME:** 10 minutes **COOK TIME:** 15 minutes

Do you like things with a little kick? Do you like chicken? Oh, you do? Then this was made just for you. When you want a burger-ish meal, but also want something a little lighter, this might just be the thing to fill that void.

1 boneless, skinless chicken breast

2 teaspoons Cajun seasoning

1 tablespoon olive oil

2 slices pepper Jack cheese

1 burger bun

1 tablespoon mayonnaise

1. Place the chicken breast on a cutting board and slice it horizontally in half, but don't go through the far side. Open it like a book.

2. Put the Cajun seasoning in a medium bowl. Add the chicken to the bowl and toss to evenly coat it.

3. Warm a medium skillet over medium-high heat. Add the olive oil and chicken and cook for about 7 minutes per side, or until the chicken is cooked through.

4. Top the chicken with the cheese and give it a minute to melt.

5. Toast the bun, then top with the mayonnaise and the chicken.

✱ **FLAVOR BOOST:** For a little extra kick, top the chicken with a few pickled jalapeños.

Per serving: Calories: 661; Total Fat: 42g; Saturated Fat: 13g; Protein: 40g; Total Carbohydrates: 29g; Fiber: 1g; Sugar: 5g; Cholesterol: 126mg

STEAK SANDWICHES

SERVES: 2 **PREP TIME:** 5 minutes, plus 40 minutes to thaw and rest
COOK TIME: 20 minutes

When cooking any steak, there are three things you need to remember. The first is to let the steak come to room temperature before cooking it so that it cooks evenly throughout. The second is to let it rest for at least 5 minutes after cooking to allow the juices to redistribute throughout the meat and to keep it juicy. The third thing to keep in mind is that, when slicing a steak, always cut across the grain. This shortens the muscle fibers and makes the meat more tender.

---

1 (6-ounce) New York strip loin steak

3 tablespoons olive oil, divided

Salt

Freshly ground black pepper

1 cup sliced onions

1 cup sliced mushrooms

1 (12-inch) baguette

2 cups baby spinach

---

1. Take the steak out of the fridge and let it sit at room temperature for 30 minutes before cooking.

2. Preheat the oven to 400°F.

3. Preheat a medium skillet over medium-high heat. Add 1 tablespoon of olive oil. Season the room-temperature steak well with salt and pepper. Add to the pan and sear for 3 minutes on each side. Take the steak out of the pan, place it on a plate, and let it rest for 5 minutes.

4. Meanwhile, return the skillet to the heat and add 1 tablespoon of oil, the onions, and mushrooms and cook for 4 to 5 minutes, or until the onions are soft and the mushrooms are lightly browned.

5. Slice the baguette horizontally in half lengthwise. Brush with the remaining 1 tablespoon olive oil and toast in the oven for 4 to 5 minutes, until lightly toasted.

6. Add the spinach to the skillet with the mushrooms and onions, season it with salt and pepper, and cook until the spinach is wilted. Remove from the heat.

7. To assemble the sandwich, lay the mushrooms and onions down on the bread first, slice the steak across the grain into ¼-inch-thick slices, and put it on top. Top the sandwich with the other slice of bread. Wrap the sandwich tightly in foil and let it sit for about 5 minutes before eating. This will soften the bread and allow all the flavors to combine.

FLAVOR BOOST: This sandwich is especially good when the baguette is brushed with a little Dijon mustard and topped with Swiss cheese.

Per serving: Calories: 676; Total Fat: 26g; Saturated Fat: 5g; Protein: 35g; Total Carbohydrates: 77g; Fiber: 5g; Sugar: 5g; Cholesterol: 42mg

CBGB (CHICKEN, BACON, GUACAMOLE, BREAD)

SERVES: 1   **PREP TIME:** 10 minutes   **COOK TIME:** 30 minutes

Named after the famous New York rock 'n' roll club, this chicken sandwich is stripped down and delicious. It's light enough that you'll feel good about eating it, but not so light that it doesn't taste good.

1 boneless, skinless chicken breast

2 slices bacon

Salt

Freshly ground black pepper

2 slices sourdough bread

2 tablespoons guacamole, homemade (page 48) or store-bought

2 slices (¼ inch thick) tomato

1. Place the chicken breast on a cutting board and slice it horizontally in half, but don't go through the far side. Open it like a book.

2. Put the bacon in a medium skillet. Set the pan over medium heat and slowly cook the bacon 5 to 6 minutes per side, until it is crispy. Take the bacon out of the pan and put it on some paper towels to drain.

3. Increase the heat to medium-high. Season the chicken with salt and pepper and cook in the pan for 6 to 7 minutes per side, until cooked through.

4. Toast the bread, then top with guacamole, tomato slices, chicken, and bacon.

✳ FLAVOR BOOST: To add a bit more punch to this sandwich, top it with pepper Jack cheese or hot sauce.

Per serving: Calories: 465; Total Fat: 12g; Saturated Fat: 3g; Protein: 40g; Total Carbohydrates: 48g; Fiber: 3g; Sugar: 5g; Cholesterol: 96mg

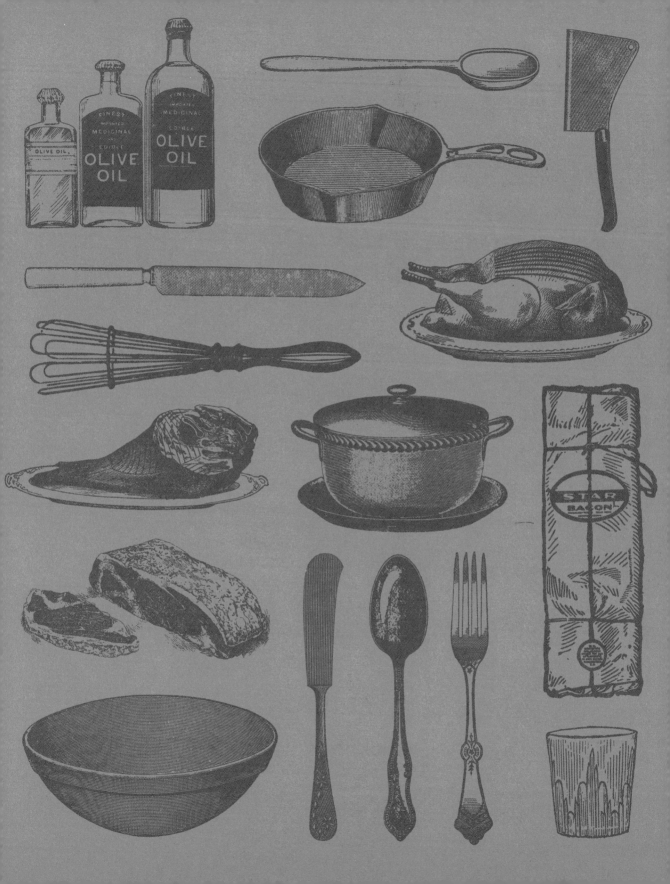

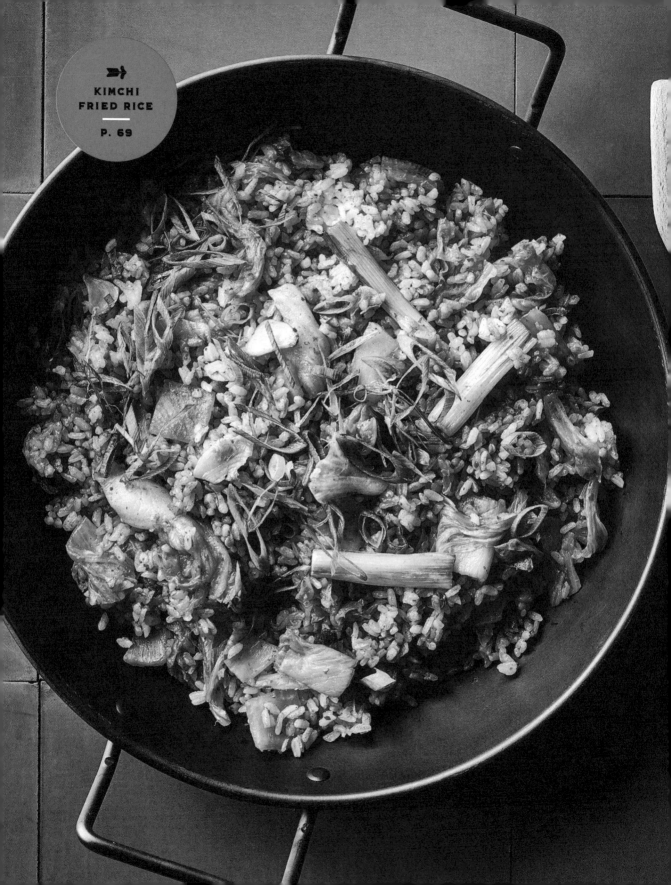

KIMCHI
FRIED RICE

P. 69

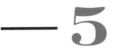

BRAWNY RICE, GRAINS, AND BEANS

QUINOA TABBOULEH

MAKES: 2 cups   **PREP TIME:** 10 minutes, plus 1 hour to chill

Tabbouleh is a Lebanese salad made of parsley, bulgur wheat, mint, and tomatoes. This version keeps close to tradition with one exception—it uses quinoa in place of the bulgur. Quinoa is easier to find and is a super grain. Serve tabbouleh as a side dish or added to wraps and salad bowls.

1 cup cooked quinoa (cooked according to package directions)

1 cup chopped fresh parsley

1 tablespoon chopped fresh mint

½ cup finely diced tomato

1 tablespoon fresh lemon juice, plus more to taste

2 tablespoons olive oil

Salt

Freshly ground black pepper

In a medium bowl, combine the quinoa, parsley, mint, tomato, lemon juice, and olive oil. Season with salt and pepper. Taste it and add a little more lemon juice if it needs it. Refrigerate the tabbouleh for 1 hour before serving.

Per serving (1 cup): Calories: 250; Total Fat: 16g; Saturated Fat: 2g; Protein: 6g; Total Carbohydrates: 24g; Fiber: 4g; Sugar: 2g; Cholesterol: 0mg

KIMCHI FRIED RICE

SERVES: 2 **PREP TIME:** 5 minutes **COOK TIME:** 10 minutes

Kimchi is a flavorful Korean condiment made of fermented cabbage and seasoning. Essentially, it's very similar to sauerkraut. Throughout its 3,000-year history, kimchi has traditionally been made at home, but it's now also widely available in most grocery stores. It's a great ingredient for adding lots of flavor with very few ingredients or effort.

4 scallions

1 tablespoon olive oil

2 garlic cloves, very thinly sliced

½ cup kimchi

1 cup cooked sticky rice, cooled completely (see A Note on Sticky Rice, page 9)

1 tablespoon soy sauce

Salt

Freshly ground black pepper

1. Cut the scallions in half to separate the dark-green tops from the whites. Cut the roots off the white parts, leaving as much of the scallion as possible, then cut the whites into 1-inch lengths and set aside. Slice the green tops as thinly as you can on a slight angle and set those aside.

2. Warm a large nonstick skillet or wok over high heat. Add the oil, scallion whites, and garlic and sauté for 1 to 2 minutes. Add the kimchi and cook for another 1 to 2 minutes.

3. Add the rice to the pan and let it cook for 1 to 2 minutes without stirring, then stir and let it sit for another 1 to 2 minutes. Pour the soy sauce into the pan and stir until it's evenly distributed.

4. Season the fried rice with salt and pepper, garnish with the sliced scallion greens, and serve.

FLAVOR BOOST: Ginger makes a great addition to this dish; sauté it along with the garlic. To fancy the dish up a bit, serve it with a sunny-side up egg over the top.

Per serving: Calories: 170; Total Fat: 7g; Saturated Fat: 1g; Protein: 4g; Total Carbohydrates: 23g; Fiber: 2g; Sugar: 2g; Cholesterol: 0mg

PORK FRIED RICE

SERVES: 2   **PREP TIME:** 5 minutes   **COOK TIME:** 10 minutes

Pork fried rice is a staple of Chinese restaurants all over North America. Now, you can make it at home and it will be even better than takeout. The secret to great fried rice to use day-old rice. Whenever you make rice, make twice as much as you need, then make fried rice the next day. Even though this recipe calls for sticky rice, you can use leftover basmati, or whatever you have.

---

1 tablespoon olive oil

½ cup small-cubed pork loin or shoulder

4 scallions, sliced, white and greens kept separate (see step 1 on page 69)

½ cup frozen peas and carrots

1 cup cooked sticky rice, cooled completely (see A Note on Sticky Rice, page 9)

2 tablespoons soy sauce

Salt

---

1. Warm a wok or large nonstick skillet over medium-high heat. Add the oil and pork to the pan. Leave the pork alone for 1 to 2 minutes, or until it is browned on the bottom. Give it a quick stir and leave it alone for another 1 to 2 minutes.

2. Throw the white bits of the scallions into the pan along with the peas and carrots and cook for 2 minutes.

3. Add the cooked rice to the pan, give it a stir, and (like the pork) leave it alone for 1 to 2 minutes. You want the rice to brown a bit on the bottom. Stir it and leave it alone for another 1 to 2 minutes.

4. Add the soy sauce and stir until it's evenly distributed.

5. Taste the rice and add a bit of salt if it needs it. Stir in the scallion greens and serve.

✳ FLAVOR BOOST: Stir-fry a beaten egg into the rice to get a more authentic takeout flavor.

Per serving: Calories: 242; Total Fat: 9g; Saturated Fat: 1g; Protein: 17g; Total Carbohydrates: 25g; Fiber: 3g; Sugar: 1g; Cholesterol: 37mg

REFRIED BEANS

SERVES: 2   **PREP TIME:** 5 minutes   **COOK TIME:** 15 minutes

Refried beans get a bad rap because most people only know them canned, but this homemade version will make you think twice. Refried beans can be served with warm tortillas, as a side dish, on burritos or tacos, or you can just eat them with a spoon. They may become one of your favorite things.

1 tablespoon olive oil

½ cup diced onion

2 teaspoons chopped garlic

2 teaspoons chili powder

**1 (15-ounce) can pinto beans, drained
and rinsed**

½ cup water

1 tablespoon fresh lime juice

Salt

Freshly ground black pepper

1. In a medium pot, heat the olive oil over medium heat. Add the onion and cook for about 5 minutes, or until soft and translucent. Add the garlic and cook for another minute. Sprinkle on the chili powder and cook for another minute.

2. Add the beans and water to the pot and bring it all to a boil. Reduce the heat to low and cook the mixture for 4 to 5 minutes, until about half the water has evaporated or been absorbed.

3. Remove the pot from the heat and mash the beans using a potato masher.

4. Mix the lime juice into the beans, give them a taste, and season them with salt and pepper as needed.

✳ FLAVOR BOOST: Add a little spice to the beans by throwing in a bit of jalapeño. You can also bulk up the flavor by adding 1 teaspoon dried oregano and ½ teaspoon ground cumin.

Per serving: Calories: 263; Total Fat: 9g; Saturated Fat: 1g; Protein: 12g; Total Carbohydrates: 38g; Fiber: 10g; Sugar: 3g; Cholesterol: 0mg

RED BEANS AND RICE

SERVES: 2   **PREP TIME:** 5 minutes   **COOK TIME:** 35 minutes

Beans and rice is a staple food for millions of people around the world. This version is influenced by Cuban and other Caribbean cuisines. You can eat this as a main course or as a side dish.

½ **cup diced bacon**

½ **cup Arborio rice**

½ **cup diced tomato**

1½ **teaspoons ground allspice**

1 **(15-ounce) can red kidney beans, drained and rinsed**

¾ cup water

Salt

Freshly ground black pepper

---

1. In a large pot with a tight-fitting lid over medium heat, cook the bacon for about 5 minutes, or until browned. Add the rice, tomato, and allspice and cook for another 2 to 3 minutes.

2. Add the beans and water and bring to a boil. Reduce the heat to low, cover, and simmer the rice for 17 minutes.

3. Remove from the heat and let it sit, with the lid on, for another 5 minutes.

4. Fluff the rice with a fork, season it with salt and pepper, and serve.

✳ FLAVOR BOOST: A bay leaf and a few sprigs of fresh thyme cooked with the rice will add a lot of extra flavor to this dish.

Per serving: Calories: 447; Total Fat: 9g; Saturated Fat: 3g; Protein: 22g; Total Carbohydrates: 71g; Fiber: 10g; Sugar: 6g; Cholesterol: 20mg

BACON AND MAPLE BAKED BEANS

MAKES: 2 cups   **PREP TIME:** 5 minutes   **COOK TIME:** 1 hour 10 minutes

Baked beans are the perfect side dish for a big breakfast or a barbecue. They are also delicious served with buttered toast. You cannot go wrong.

½ cup diced bacon

2 tablespoons tomato paste

1 teaspoon mustard powder

1 (15-ounce) can navy beans, drained and rinsed

¼ cup maple syrup

1 cup water

½ teaspoon salt, plus more to taste

½ teaspoon black pepper, plus more to taste

1. Preheat the oven to 325°F.

2. While the oven preheats, warm a medium Dutch oven or other oven-proof pot over medium heat. Add the bacon and cook for 4 to 5 minutes, until it's browned and crispy.

3. Add the tomato paste and cook for 1 to 2 minutes. Add the mustard powder and cook for another 30 seconds.

4. Add the beans, maple syrup, water, salt, and pepper. Bring to a boil, cover, and throw into the oven for 1 hour.

5. Remove from the oven, taste the beans, and season with salt and pepper if they need it.

Per serving (1 cup): Calories: 437; Total Fat: 8g; Saturated Fat: 3g; Protein: 21g; Total Carbohydrates: 72g; Fiber: 18g; Sugar: 27g; Cholesterol: 20mg

DAL

SERVES: 2 **PREP TIME:** 5 minutes **COOK TIME:** 40 minutes

Dal is an Indian dish made with dried split lentils. Typically, it has 10 to 20 different spices in it. Using curry powder, you can make a good-tasting dal without a thousand ingredients. On top of being delicious, dal is good for you, packs in lots of flavor, and is easy to make. Serve the dal by itself as a side dish or with rice or naan bread.

2 tablespoons olive oil

½ cup diced onion

1 tablespoon grated fresh ginger

1 tablespoon tomato paste

1 tablespoon yellow curry powder

½ cup dried red lentils

3 cups water

Salt

Freshly ground black pepper

1. Warm a medium pot over medium heat. Add the olive oil and onion and cook for 5 minutes, or until soft. Add the ginger and cook for 30 seconds. Add the tomato paste and cook for 1 minute.

2. Sprinkle the curry powder into the pot and cook for 30 seconds. Add the lentils and water and bring to a boil. Reduce the heat to low and simmer for 25 to 30 minutes, until the lentils are tender.

3. Taste the dal and add salt and pepper if it needs it.

Per serving: Calories: 330; Total Fat: 15g; Saturated Fat: 2g; Protein: 13g; Total Carbohydrates: 39g; Fiber: 8g; Sugar: 3g; Cholesterol: 0mg

BRAISED LENTILS

SERVES: 2   **PREP TIME:** 5 minutes   **COOK TIME:** 40 minutes

Braised lentils make a fantastic side dish for pork, fish, or sausages. And they come together very quickly. Dried lentils, unlike dried beans, don't need to be soaked before cooking. Just give them a quick rinse and they're good to go.

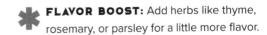

2 tablespoons olive oil

½ cup diced onion

¼ cup diced carrot

¼ cup diced celery

¼ cup white wine or vegetable broth

½ cup dried red or green lentils

2 cups water

Salt

Freshly ground black pepper

1. Warm a medium pot over medium heat. Add the olive oil, onion, carrot, and celery and cook the vegetables for 5 to 6 minutes, until the onions are translucent and the carrots are soft. Make sure to give them a shake or stir every minute or so.

2. Add the wine and cook for another 2 minutes.

3. Add the lentils and water to the pot, bring to a boil, then reduce to a simmer and cook for 30 minutes, or until the lentils are tender.

4. Season the lentils with salt and pepper and serve with your favorite protein.

✱ FLAVOR BOOST: Add herbs like thyme, rosemary, or parsley for a little more flavor.

Per serving: Calories: 343; Total Fat: 15g; Saturated Fat: 2g; Protein: 12g; Total Carbohydrates: 38g; Fiber: 7g; Sugar: 3g; Cholesterol: 0mg

CREAMY POLENTA

SERVES: 2 **PREP TIME:** 5 minutes **COOK TIME:** 25 minutes

Polenta is essentially a savory porridge commonly made of cornmeal. The technique for making polenta dates all the way back to ancient Rome—you take a grain (in this case, corn), dry it, grind it, and boil it in water until it's soft and thick. Serve this by itself or topped with Mushroom Ragu (page 82).

2 cups vegetable broth

1 bay leaf

¼ cup cornmeal

2 tablespoons salted butter

¼ cup grated Parmesan cheese

Salt

Freshly ground black pepper

1. In a medium pot, combine the broth and bay leaf and bring to a boil.

2. Whisk the cornmeal into the boiling water, reduce the heat to medium, and cook, stirring pretty much nonstop, for 15 to 20 minutes, until it has the consistency of scrambled eggs.

3. Remove the polenta from the heat and stir in the butter and Parmesan. Season the polenta with salt and pepper. Eat it as it is or serve it as a side dish.

Per serving: Calories: 224; Total Fat: 16g; Saturated Fat: 9g; Protein: 5g; Total Carbohydrates: 17g; Fiber: 1g; Sugar: 2g; Cholesterol: 41mg

RISOTTO BASE

SERVES: 2 **PREP TIME:** 5 minutes **COOK TIME:** 25 minutes

Risotto is an Italian dish made with a special kind of starchy rice. The rice is cooked slowly and stirred constantly as liquid is added. This technique draws the starch out of the rice, making the risotto creamy without ever adding cream. This risotto base is just that: a base. It's not meant to be eaten as is, but to be added to. You can use it to make Pea and Prosciutto Risotto (page 78), Chicken and Mushroom Risotto (page 79), or add beets, seafood, and just about anything else you can think of.

4 cups chicken stock

1 tablespoon olive oil

¼ cup minced onion

1 teaspoon minced garlic

½ cup Arborio rice

¼ cup white wine

Salt

Freshly ground black pepper

1. In a medium pot, bring the stock to a boil. Reduce the heat to low so that the stock remains hot.

2. Warm a medium saucepan over medium heat. Add the olive oil, onion, and garlic and cook for 1 minute.

3. Add the rice to the pan and cook for 1 minute, then add the wine and cook until it has just about completely evaporated.

4. Add a ladleful of stock. Stir the rice and cook until the stock has been almost completely absorbed by the rice. Repeat this process until the rice is tender and creamy and all the stock has been used. It should take about 20 minutes.

5. Season the risotto with salt and pepper and garnish it with whatever other ingredients you want.

✳ **SUBSTITUTION TIP:** If you can't find Arborio rice, use Carnaroli rice instead. It may be labeled as "risotto rice" at the grocery store.

Per serving: Calories: 296; Total Fat: 7g; Saturated Fat: 1g; Protein: 12g; Total Carbohydrates: 41g; Fiber: 2g; Sugar: 1g; Cholesterol: 0mg

PEA AND PROSCIUTTO RISOTTO

SERVES: 2 **PREP TIME:** 5 minutes **COOK TIME:** 25 minutes

The white wine in the risotto base adds a slight acidity to the rice. When combined with the sweetness of peas and the salty umami flavor of prosciutto, that acidity is perfectly balanced. This is a dish that you'll try once and then crave for every special occasion.

Risotto Base (page 77)

¼ cup frozen peas

1 tablespoon olive oil

2 slices prosciutto, cut into thin strips

2 tablespoons grated Parmesan cheese

1 tablespoon salted butter

---

1. Make the risotto base as directed, but just before adding the last bit of stock, add the frozen peas.

2. Meanwhile, in a small skillet, heat the olive oil and prosciutto and cook over medium heat until the prosciutto is crisp.

3. Drain the crisp prosciutto in a sieve to get rid of the oil, then stir into the cooked risotto. Finish the risotto by stirring in the Parmesan and butter.

Per serving: Calories: 402; Total Fat: 16g; Saturated Fat: 6g; Protein: 17g; Total Carbohydrates: 44g; Fiber: 3g; Sugar: 2g; Cholesterol: 26mg

CHICKEN AND MUSHROOM RISOTTO

SERVES: 2   **PREP TIME:** 5 minutes   **COOK TIME:** 50 minutes

Chicken and mushroom risotto is the perfect thing to make when you have a guest coming over, want to impress your mom, or just want to treat yourself to something special. This takes some time to make because you have to cook the chicken, but it's definitely worth the effort.

2 bone-in, skin-on chicken thighs
Salt
Freshly ground black pepper
1 tablespoon olive oil
½ cup sliced cremini mushrooms
2 tablespoons butter, divided
Risotto Base (page 77)
2 tablespoons grated Parmesan cheese

1. Preheat the oven to 400°F.

2. Pat the chicken thighs dry with paper towels and season them well with salt and pepper.

3. Warm an ovenproof medium skillet over medium-high heat. Add the olive oil and place the chicken in the pan skin-side down. Let it cook for 4 to 5 minutes. The skin should be well browned and crispy before it is flipped.

4. Flip the chicken and cook for 2 more minutes. Add the mushrooms to the pan along with 1 tablespoon of butter. Put the whole thing in the oven for 15 to 20 minutes, until the chicken is cooked through.

5. Using a fork, take the crispy skin off the chicken, chop it into small pieces and set it aside. Using two forks, pull the chicken off the bones and cut it into small pieces.

6. Make the risotto base as directed. Once the risotto is cooked, add the chicken, mushrooms, Parmesan, and remaining 1 tablespoon butter.

7. Finish the risotto by crumbling the crispy chicken skin over the top.

Per serving: Calories: 915; Total Fat: 59g; Saturated Fat: 19g; Protein: 47g; Total Carbohydrates: 44g; Fiber: 3g; Sugar: 2g; Cholesterol: 225mg

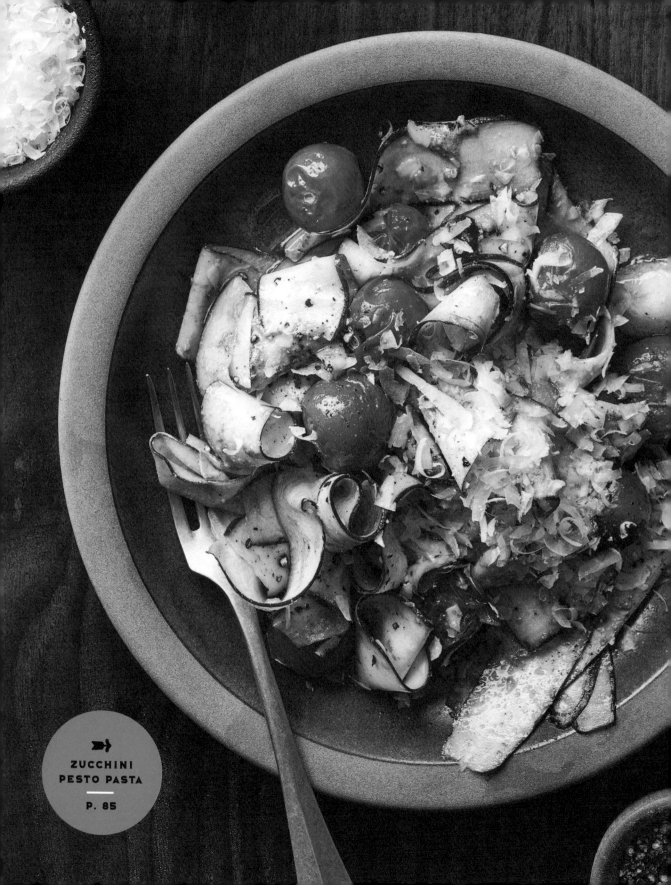

ZUCCHINI
PESTO PASTA

P. 85

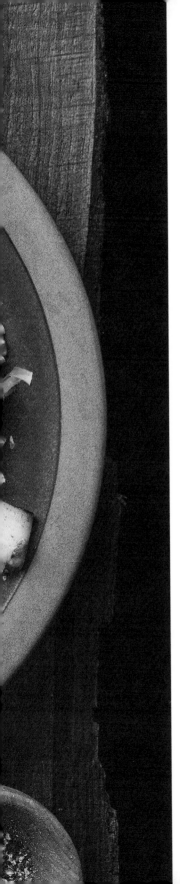

6

POTENT PLANT-BASED EATS

MUSHROOM RAGU

SERVES: 4   **PREP TIME:** 5 minutes   **COOK TIME:** 30 minutes

Ragu is a classic Italian pasta sauce containing tomato and meat. This version substitutes mushrooms for the meat and adds red wine to deepen the flavor. Serve this on your favorite pasta or on Creamy Polenta (page 76).

---

2 tablespoons olive oil

2 cups sliced cremini mushrooms

½ cup diced onion

2 tablespoons tomato paste

½ cup red wine

1 cup water

1 tablespoon chopped rosemary

Salt

Freshly ground black pepper

---

1. Warm a medium pot over medium heat. Add the olive oil, mushrooms, and onion and cook 5 to 8 minutes, until the onion is soft and the mushrooms are cooked through.

2. Add the tomato paste and cook for another 2 to 3 minutes, stirring constantly.

3. Add the red wine and cook for 2 minutes. Add the water and rosemary and simmer the sauce for 15 minutes, or until thick. Season with salt and pepper.

Per serving: Calories: 112; Total Fat: 7g; Saturated Fat: 1g; Protein: 2g; Total Carbohydrates: 7g; Fiber: 1g; Sugar: 3g; Cholesterol: 0mg

MUSHROOM AND GOAT CHEESE PASTA

SERVES: 2 **PREP TIME:** 5 minutes **COOK TIME:** 25 minutes

To make the flavors of this simple pasta dish pop, buy a pack of mixed mushrooms at the grocery store. These packs will generally contain cremini or button mushrooms, portobello, and possibly oyster mushrooms. If you can't find a pack of mixed mushrooms, buy a couple of different mushrooms individually.

2 cups evenly sliced mixed mushrooms

2 tablespoons olive oil

Salt

Freshly ground black pepper

4 ounces dried fettuccine

2 tablespoons salted butter

6 sage leaves

¼ cup crumbled goat cheese

1. Preheat the oven to 400°F. Line a baking sheet with parchment paper.

2. In a medium bowl, toss the mushrooms with the olive oil and a bit of salt and pepper. Spread the mushrooms out on the lined baking sheet and roast in the oven for 15 to 20 minutes.

3. While the mushrooms are baking, cook the pasta according to the package directions.

4. While the pasta is cooking, warm a medium skillet over medium heat. Add the butter and, once it starts to bubble, add the sage leaves. Cook for 1 minute, or until the leaves start to crisp. Add the mushrooms, goat cheese, and 2 tablespoons of water from the pasta pot.

5. Remove the skillet from the heat and stir the sauce together. Drain the pasta, toss it in the sauce, and season it with salt and pepper.

✳ SUBSTITUTION TIP: You can substitute 6 ounces fresh fettuccine for the dried.

Per serving: Calories: 612; Total Fat: 40g; Saturated Fat: 19g; Protein: 20g; Total Carbohydrates: 45g; Fiber: 3g; Sugar: 3g; Cholesterol: 66mg

PASTA PRIMAVERA

SERVES: 2 **PREP TIME:** 5 minutes **COOK TIME:** 15 minutes

Pasta primavera is a pasta dish loaded with fresh seasonal vegetables and tossed with tomato sauce. In this version the sauce is a mushroom ragu, which gives the pasta a little more flavor and depth than the traditional marinara sauce does.

4 ounces (1⅓ cups) penne pasta

2 tablespoons olive oil

½ cup sliced red bell pepper

½ cup broccoli florets

1 tablespoon chopped garlic

1 cup Mushroom Ragu (page 82)

Salt

Freshly ground black pepper

1. Cook the pasta according to the package directions.

2. While the pasta is cooking, warm a medium skillet over medium-high heat. Add the olive oil, bell peppers, and broccoli and cook for 5 minutes, stirring every minute or so, until the vegetables begin to soften.

3. Add the garlic to the pan and cook for 45 seconds to 1 minute, just until it starts to turn golden brown. Add the mushroom ragu sauce. Cook for 5 to 6 minutes, until the sauce is hot and the vegetables are tender. You may need to stir a few tablespoons of the pasta cooking water into the sauce if it starts to get too thick.

4. Toss the pasta into the sauce, season with salt and pepper, and serve.

✳ **FLAVOR BOOST:** Any kind of fresh vegetable can be added to this pasta. Use what is freshest at the grocery store or market.

Per serving: Calories: 621; Total Fat: 18g; Saturated Fat: 3g; Protein: 17g; Total Carbohydrates: 98g; Fiber: 6g; Sugar: 11g; Cholesterol: 0mg

ZUCCHINI PESTO PASTA

SERVES: 1   **PREP TIME:** 5 minutes   **COOK TIME:** 10 minutes

This recipe is based around noodles made from zucchini. You can use a spiralizer to make the noodles if you have one, or you can shave the zucchini into long wide noodles using a vegetable peeler.

1 cup zucchini noodles

2 tablespoons water

1 tablespoon olive oil

12 cherry tomatoes

2 tablespoons pesto, homemade (page 149) or store-bought

Salt

Freshly ground black pepper

2 tablespoons grated Parmesan cheese

1. Put the zucchini noodles in a microwave-safe dish along with the water. Cover the dish tightly with plastic wrap and cook in the microwave on high for 90 seconds.

2. Warm a medium skillet over medium-high heat. Add the olive oil and cherry tomatoes and cook the tomatoes until they start to pop, about 3 to 4 minutes.

3. Add the zucchini noodles, along with the cooking water, to the pan. Add the pesto, toss, season with salt and pepper, and finish with the Parmesan.

✳ **FLAVOR BOOST:** If you would like to bulk this dish up or add a little more protein, you can add a cooked and sliced chicken breast. In addition to the chicken, or alternatively, you can add cooked and diced bacon.

Per serving: Calories: 373; Total Fat: 34g; Saturated Fat: 6g; Protein: 7g; Total Carbohydrates: 13g; Fiber: 4g; Sugar: 7g; Cholesterol: 12mg

MISO BLACK BEAN BURGER PATTIES

SERVES: 4   **PREP TIME:** 10 minutes   **COOK TIME:** 25 minutes

Miso is a Japanese fermented soybean paste. You can find it at most grocery or specialty stores. The miso in this recipe gives the black bean burger that "meaty" umami flavor that's often missing with vegetable burgers. All that to say that this is a vegetable burger you'll actually enjoy eating. Throw the patties on a bun, top with your favorite ingredients, and you're good to go.

1 (15-ounce) can black beans, drained and rinsed

2 teaspoons miso paste

½ teaspoon onion powder

½ teaspoon garlic powder

¼ cup fine dried bread crumbs

¼ teaspoon salt

¼ teaspoon freshly ground black pepper

2 tablespoons water

1. Preheat the oven to 350°F. Line a baking sheet with parchment paper.

2. Pat the black beans dry with paper towels and put them in a food processor. Add the miso, onion powder, garlic powder, bread crumbs, salt, pepper, and water and pulse until the mixture comes together and is sticky.

3. Divide the black bean mixture into 4 even portions and form into patties. Place the patties on the lined baking sheet and bake for 22 minutes, flipping about halfway through, until lightly golden on both sides.

4. Remove the patties from the oven and serve or let cool. If you are serving them later, reheat them in a hot pan with a bit of oil.

PREP TIP: If you don't have a food processor, you can mash all the ingredients together using a potato masher.

Per serving: Calories: 139; Total Fat: 1g; Saturated Fat: <1g; Protein: 8g; Total Carbohydrates: 25g; Fiber: 8g; Sugar: 1g; Cholesterol: 0mg

PORTOBELLO MUSHROOM BURGER

SERVES: 1 **PREP TIME:** 5 minutes **COOK TIME:** 10 minutes

Portobello mushrooms naturally have a meaty taste and texture. Pan-roast them, top them with cheese, throw them inside a bun with some garlic mayo, and you have a burger that can't be beat even by meat.

1 tablespoon olive oil

1 (4- to 5-inch) portobello mushroom

Salt

Freshly ground black pepper

¼ cup shredded mozzarella cheese

1 burger bun

2 tablespoons mayonnaise

½ teaspoon garlic powder

1. Cut off and discard the stem from the mushroom.

2. Warm a small skillet over medium-high heat. Add the oil and the mushroom to the pan stemmed-side down. Season with salt and pepper, then put a lid on the pan and let the mushroom cook for 4 minutes. Flip the mushroom and cook for 4 more minutes. Put the mozzarella on the mushroom, cover the pan again and cook for 1 minute to melt the cheese.

3. While the mushroom is cooking, toast the bun and mix the mayonnaise and garlic powder together.

4. Spread the garlic mayo on the bun, top with the mushroom, and enjoy.

PREP TIP: The mushroom can also be grilled or oven-roasted on 400°F for 20 minutes. A grilled mushroom will take on a light smoky flavor, while an oven-roasted mushroom will be more evenly cooked than either grilled or pan-roasted.

Per serving: Calories: 535; Total Fat: 43g; Saturated Fat: 10g; Protein: 12g; Total Carbohydrates: 26g; Fiber: 2g; Sugar: 6g; Cholesterol: 37mg

MEATLESS MEATLOAF

SERVES: 6   **PREP TIME:** 15 minutes, plus 10 minutes to rest
COOK TIME: 1 hour 30 minutes

This meatless meatloaf is delicious and good for you. Lentils make a good textural substitute for ground beef, and the mushrooms add that meaty flavor that is missing from vegetarian dishes. If you're looking for something a little different and a little lighter than a traditional meatloaf, you've found just the thing.

1 cup dried lentils

3 cups water

2 teaspoons olive oil

½ cup minced onion

2 cups chopped mushrooms

2 tablespoons minced garlic

1 teaspoon salt

¼ teaspoon freshly ground black pepper

½ cup whole-milk Greek yogurt

Per serving: Calories: 147; Total Fat: 3g; Saturated Fat: 1g; Protein: 9g; Total Carbohydrates: 21g; Fiber: 5g; Sugar: 3g; Cholesterol: 3mg

1. Preheat the oven to 350°F.

2. Rinse the lentils, put them in a medium pot, and add the water. Bring to a boil, then reduce the heat to low and simmer the lentils for 25 to 30 minutes, until they are tender. Remove from the heat and let the lentils sit for another 10 minutes.

3. Drain the lentils in a sieve, transfer to a food processor, and puree. (Or mash in a bowl with a potato masher.) Set aside.

4. Warm a medium skillet over medium heat. Add the olive oil and onion to the pan and cook for 5 minutes. Add the mushrooms, garlic, salt, and pepper. Reduce the heat to medium-low and cook for 8 to 10 minutes, until all the moisture has been cooked out of the mushrooms.

5. Remove from the heat and transfer the mushrooms and onions to the food processor with the lentils. Add the yogurt and puree.

6. Put the mixture into an 8½-by-4½-inch loaf pan, and pat down to pack it in tightly. Cover with aluminum foil and bake for 45 minutes.

7. Leave the loaf in the pan and let cool for 10 minutes before slicing and serving.

TOFU NOODLE BOWLS

SERVES: 4 **PREP TIME:** 5 minutes, plus 30 minutes to soak **COOK TIME:** 10 minutes

This simple soup is great on a crisp autumn day, a cold winter day, a warm spring day, or a beautiful summer day. Yeah, it's good all the time. Even though there isn't much to it, it's filling and packs a lot of flavor. Serve the soup with sambal or sriracha on the side.

8 cups water

1 cup dried shiitake mushrooms

¼ cup soy sauce

1 tablespoon cornstarch

1 (14-ounce) package tofu, diced

1 teaspoon salt

¼ teaspoon freshly ground black pepper

8 ounces dried rice noodles, cooked according to package directions

1. In a large pot, combine the water and dried mushrooms. Let the mushrooms soak for 30 minutes.

2. Take the mushrooms out of the water and cut into ⅛-inch-thick slices. Return the mushrooms to the pot and bring the water to a boil over high heat.

3. In a small bowl, stir the soy sauce and cornstarch together and add to the soup along with the tofu. Bring the soup to a boil, then reduce the heat to low and simmer for 5 minutes.

4. Season the soup with the salt and pepper. Divide the noodles among four bowls, ladle the broth over the noodles, and enjoy.

✳ FLAVOR BOOST: Vegetables such as carrots, bok choy, spinach, onion, and garlic can be added to the soup to give it more flavor and substance.

Per serving: Calories: 338; Total Fat: 5g; Saturated Fat: 1g; Protein: 15g; Total Carbohydrates: 56g; Fiber: 2g; Sugar: 1g; Cholesterol: 0mg

ROASTED VEGETABLES

SERVES: 4 **PREP TIME:** 10 minutes **COOK TIME:** 32 minutes

Roasted vegetables make the perfect side dish, snack, or salad when tossed with lettuce and dressing. Not only are these roasted vegetables delicious, but they're also versatile. Use whatever vegetables are in season, mix and match, and enjoy. Oh, and don't worry too much about the measurements. For something like this, it really doesn't matter that much because having a little more red bell pepper or a little less onion isn't going change the flavor or cooking time.

½ **cup diced zucchini**

12 cherry tomatoes

½ **cup diced red bell pepper**

½ **cup diced red onion**

½ **cup diced sweet potato**

2 tablespoons olive oil

Salt

Freshly ground black pepper

1. Preheat the oven to 400°F. Line a sheet pan with parchment paper.

2. In a large bowl, combine the zucchini, tomatoes, bell pepper, onion, and sweet potato. Add the olive oil and season with salt and pepper. Stir or toss to mix evenly.

3. Spread the vegetables out on the lined sheet pan. Roast them in the oven for 12 minutes, flip them over, and continue roasting for 15–20 minutes longer, until they're tender.

Per serving: Calories: 115; Total Fat: 7g; Saturated Fat: 1g; Protein: 2g; Total Carbohydrates: 13g; Fiber: 3g; Sugar: 5g; Cholesterol: 0mg

ROASTED SWEET POTATO FINGERS

SERVES: 2   **PREP TIME:** 5 minutes   **COOK TIME:** 35 minutes

Inspired by a sushi roll, these sweet potato fingers with sweet soy glaze and guacamole are guaranteed to please. They make a great snack or the perfect thing for your next Super Bowl party. It may seem like a strange combination when you read the recipe, but do yourself a favor and try it.

---

1 fist-size sweet potato

2 tablespoons olive oil

Freshly ground black pepper

¼ cup soy sauce

3 tablespoons sugar

Salt

½ cup guacamole, homemade (page 48) or
  store-bought

---

1. Preheat the oven to 375°F.

2. Peel the sweet potato and cut it into finger-size pieces. Put the fingers in a large bowl, drizzle with olive oil, and season with pepper. Toss to evenly coat the fingers.

3. Spread the sweet potato fingers out onto a sheet pan and roast for 20 minutes. Flip the sweet potatoes and roast for another 10 to 15 minutes, until they are tender.

4. While the potato fingers are cooking, in a small pot, combine soy sauce and sugar and bring to a boil. Reduce the heat to a simmer and cook about 5 minutes, or until thick. Remove from the heat and let cool.

5. Take the sweet potatoes out of the oven, season with salt, drizzle with the sweet soy glaze, and serve with guacamole on the side.

Per serving: Calories: 302; Total Fat: 17g; Saturated Fat: 2g; Protein: 4g; Total Carbohydrates: 37g; Fiber: 4g; Sugar: 22g; Cholesterol: 0mg

CREAMY GARLIC MASHED POTATOES

    VG

SERVES: 4 **PREP TIME:** 10 minutes **COOK TIME:** 20 minutes

Who doesn't love mashed potatoes? People who haven't had these mashed potatoes, that's who. Serve these potatoes with just about anything and the meal will become instantly memorable. These pair especially well with Meatless Meatloaf (page 88).

---

3 cups diced peeled yellow potatoes
Salt
3 garlic cloves, peeled
¼ cup heavy cream
2 tablespoons salted butter
Freshly ground black pepper

---

1. In a medium pot, add the potatoes with enough water to cover them. Add a pinch of salt. Bring to a boil over high heat and boil for 5 minutes. Add the whole cloves of garlic and continue to cook until the potatoes are tender, approximately 15 minutes.

2. Drain the potatoes in a colander. Let them sit in the colander for at least 3 minutes to steam-dry.

3. While the potatoes are sitting, put the cream and butter in the potato pot along with some salt and pepper. Heat the cream and butter just until the butter melts.

4. Return the potatoes and garlic to the pot and mash with a potato masher until smooth. Taste the potatoes and season with a little more salt and pepper if needed.

✳ **PREP TIP:** Use a food mill instead of a masher to get extra smooth and creamy potatoes.

Per serving: Calories: 184; Total Fat: 11g; Saturated Fat: 7g; Protein: 3g; Total Carbohydrates: 19g; Fiber: 2g; Sugar: 2g; Cholesterol: 32mg

CAULIFLOWER RICE

SERVES: 4   **PREP TIME:** 10 minutes   **COOK TIME:** 15 minutes

If you're trying to cut back on carbs, there isn't a much better side dish than cauliflower rice. It helps that it's easy and quick to make. Cauliflower rice makes a great side for stir-fries, curry, or just about anything.

---

1 head cauliflower, leaves and stem trimmed off
1 tablespoon olive oil
Salt
Freshly ground black pepper
1 tablespoon salted butter

---

1. Grate the cauliflower on the large holes of a box grater into a large bowl.

2. Warm a large skillet with a lid over medium-high heat. Add the olive oil and cauliflower and cook for 3 to 4 minutes, until the cauliflower looks wet.

3. Cover the pan and remove from the heat. Let the cauliflower sit for 10 minutes. Season it with salt and pepper, and add the butter. Fluff it with a fork and serve.

✱ PREP TIP: To make the cauliflower rice more quickly, you can pulse the cauliflower in a food processor a few times instead of grating it. The pieces won't be as evenly sized, but it will save time.

Per serving: Calories: 92; Total Fat: 7g; Saturated Fat: 3g; Protein: 3g; Total Carbohydrates: 7g; Fiber: 3g; Sugar: 3g; Cholesterol: 8mg

VEGETABLE STIR-FRY

SERVES: 2   **PREP TIME:** 10 minutes   **COOK TIME:** 15 minutes

There's very little that beats a stir-fry for speed, convenience, and deliciousness. With this recipe, you'll have a great meal that you can feel good about because you're eating all of these vegetables and they taste amazing.

2 tablespoons olive oil

½ cup sliced onion

½ cup sliced carrot

½ cup sliced green bell pepper

1 cup bean sprouts, rinsed and patted dry

¾ cup stir-fry sauce, homemade (page 151) or store-bought

Salt

Freshly ground black pepper

1. Warm a large skillet over medium-high heat. Add the oil, onion, and carrot and cook for 4 minutes, stirring every 30 seconds.

2. Add the bell pepper and cook for another 2 minutes. Add the bean sprouts and cook for 3 more minutes.

3. Pour in the sauce and cook for 2 more minutes, or until thick. Taste and season with salt and pepper.

FLAVOR BOOST: You can add any fresh vegetable you'd like into this stir-fry. Additionally, you can add tofu for a kick of protein.

Per serving: Calories: 231; Total Fat: 14g; Saturated Fat: 2g; Protein: 5g; Total Carbohydrates: 25g; Fiber: 3g; Sugar: 15g; Cholesterol: 0mg

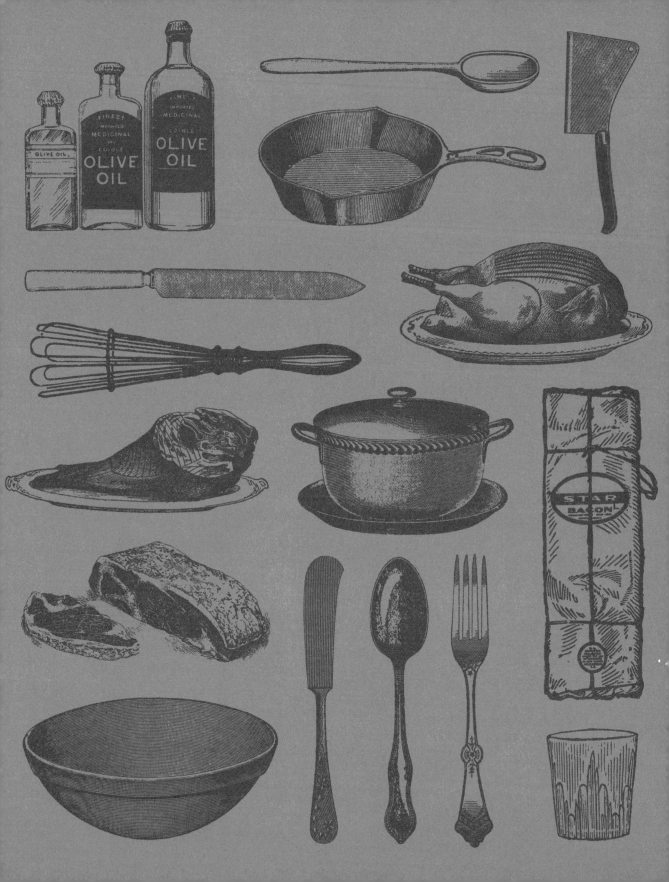

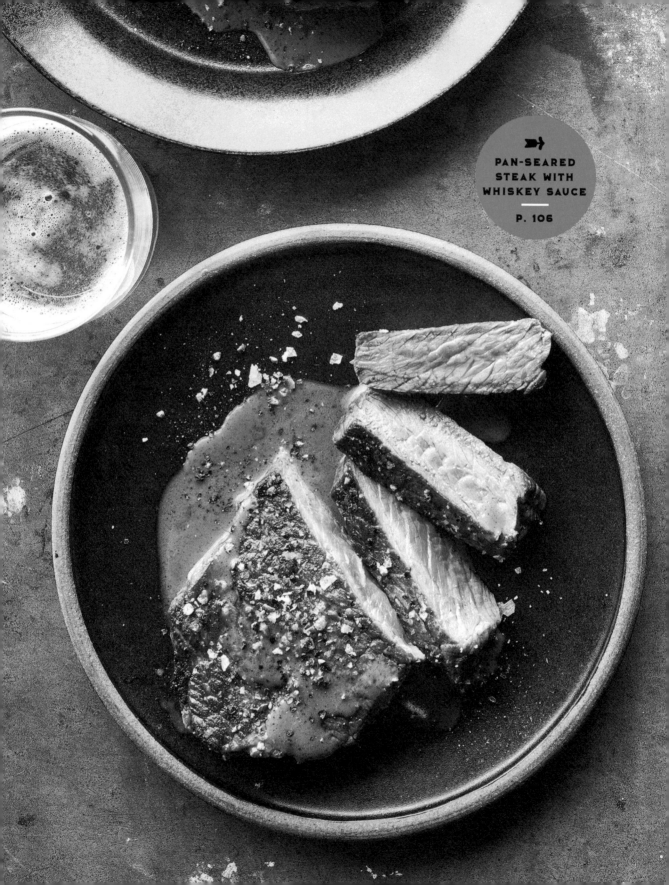

PAN-SEARED STEAK WITH WHISKEY SAUCE

P. 106

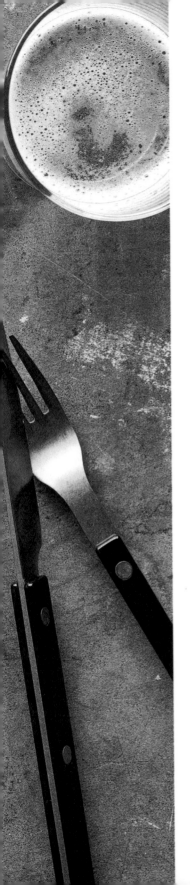

7

MANLY MEAT AND POULTRY MAINS

MOM'S SHEPHERD'S PIE

SERVES: 6   **PREP TIME:** 10 minutes, plus 20 minutes to rest   **COOK TIME:** 1 hour

There are few things more comforting in the world than a big plate of shepherd's pie. Though traditionally made with lamb, this version uses ground beef, just the way Mom used to make it. Rather than making a gravy, the cream-style corn creates a thick and creamy sauce that perfectly balances the savory, meaty flavor.

1 tablespoon olive oil

1 pound medium ground beef

1 cup diced onion

2 cups frozen vegetable medley (peas, carrots, green beans)

2 (14.75-ounce) cans cream-style corn

Salt

Freshly ground black pepper

Creamy Garlic Mashed Potatoes (page 92), doubled recipe

1. Preheat the oven to 375°F.

2. Warm a large ovenproof skillet over medium-high heat. Add the olive oil and ground beef. Cook the beef for 9 to 10 minutes, until it is browned.

3. Drain off the fat, add the onion to the pan, and cook for another 5 minutes. Add the frozen vegetable medley and cook for another 3 to 4 minutes to warm the vegetables.

4. Add the cream-style corn and cook just until it starts to boil. Taste the mixture and season it with salt and pepper. Remove from the heat, smooth out the top using a spatula, and let it rest for 10 minutes.

5. Cover the shepherd's pie with the mashed potatoes. Put the skillet on a baking sheet and bake in the oven for 35 minutes. Remove from the oven and let the shepherd's pie rest for another 10 minutes before serving.

Per serving: Calories: 569; Total Fat: 30g; Saturated Fat: 15g; Protein: 22g; Total Carbohydrates: 57g; Fiber: 6g; Sugar: 10g; Cholesterol: 88mg

BEEF AND BROCCOLI

SERVES: 2   **PREP TIME:** 5 minutes   **COOK TIME:** 15 minutes

Beef and broccoli is a Chinese takeout staple for a reason: It's delicious. Now, you can make it at home and enjoy it whenever you'd like.

3 tablespoons olive oil, divided

½ pound flank steak, thinly sliced across the grain

Salt

Freshly ground black pepper

1 cup broccoli florets

2 tablespoons water

½ cup sliced onion

1 tablespoon sliced garlic

¾ cup stir-fry sauce, homemade (page 151) or store-bought

1. Warm a medium skillet over medium-high heat. Add 1 tablespoon of olive oil and the steak. Season the steak with salt and pepper. Cook only until browned, about 3–5 minutes. Take the steak out of the pan and set aside.

2. Set the skillet back over medium-high heat. Add 1 tablespoon of oil and the broccoli and sauté the broccoli for 2 minutes. Add the water to the pan, cover, and steam the broccoli for 2 minutes. Take the broccoli out of the pan and set aside.

3. Wipe the pan out with a paper towel and return it to the heat. Add the remaining 1 tablespoon of oil along with the onion. Cook until onions are soft, about 3 minutes. Then, return the cooked steak to the pot.

4. Add the garlic and cook for 1 more minute. Return the broccoli to the pan along with the stir-fry sauce and cook for 2 more minutes.

5. Taste the stir-fry and season with salt and pepper as needed.

Per serving: Calories: 401; Total Fat: 23g; Saturated Fat: 6g; Protein: 28g; Total Carbohydrates: 21g; Fiber: 2g; Sugar: 11g; Cholesterol: 53mg

CHICKEN AND MUSHROOM STIR-FRY

SERVES: 2 **PREP TIME:** 5 minutes **COOK TIME:** 12 minutes

The secret to a good stir-fry is maintaining the heat of the pan or wok. If the pan cools down too much, all the moisture coming out of the vegetables and meat will get stuck and pool in the bottom of the pan. This will boil your ingredients and make them soggy as opposed to the crisp vegetables and tender meat that are hallmarks of a good stir-fry. Don't be afraid to use medium-high to high heat to cook this stir-fry. Make sure to stir or toss the ingredients every 15 to 30 seconds. It's called a *stir*-fry, after all. Serve this with rice or Cauliflower Rice (page 93).

1. Warm a large skillet or wok over medium-high heat. Add the oil and chicken and cook for 4 to 5 minutes, until the chicken is browned.

2. Add the mushrooms, onion, and garlic and cook for 4 to 5 minutes, stirring the ingredients every minute or so, until the onion and garlic just start to brown.

3. Add the sauce to the pan and cook for another 1 to 2 minutes, until the sauce is thick. Remove from the heat, taste the sauce, and season with salt and pepper.

＊ SUBSTITUTION TIP: You can use ¾ cup store-bought sesame-ginger stir-fry sauce in place of the homemade sauce here.

---

1 tablespoon olive oil

1 boneless, skinless chicken breast, thinly sliced

½ cup quartered mushrooms

½ cup sliced onion

1 tablespoon sliced garlic

¾ cup stir-fry sauce, homemade (page 151) or store-bought

Salt

Freshly ground black pepper

Per serving: Calories: 212; Total Fat: 9g; Saturated Fat: 1g; Protein: 16g; Total Carbohydrates: 19g; Fiber: 1g; Sugar: 11g; Cholesterol: 40mg

CAVEMAN ROASTED TURKEY LEGS

SERVES: 2 **PREP TIME:** 5 minutes **COOK TIME:** 1 hour

Every man has a bit of caveman in him. And even though you won't be walking around munching on mammoth ribs any time soon, it doesn't mean that you can't get in touch with your caveman roots every once in a while. These tasty turkey legs are a little sweet, a little smoky, and will make your caveman ancestors proud. For a little extra punch of flavor, brush the legs with a little All-Purpose BBQ Sauce (page 152).

1 teaspoon light brown sugar

1 teaspoon garlic powder

1 teaspoon onion powder

1 teaspoon smoked paprika

1 teaspoon salt

1 teaspoon freshly ground black pepper

2 turkey drumsticks

2 teaspoons olive oil

1. Preheat the oven to 375°F.

2. In a small bowl, stir together the brown sugar, garlic powder, onion powder, smoked paprika, salt, and pepper.

3. Season the turkey drumsticks generously with the seasoning blend. Use the oil to lightly coat a small roasting pan. Put the drumsticks in the pan, making sure they aren't touching, and roast them for 30 minutes.

4. Flip the turkey legs and roast for another 30 minutes, or until a thermometer inserted into the thickest part of the meat registers 170°F.

SUBSTITUTION TIP: You can substitute chicken legs for the turkey legs, but cut the total cooking time down by about 15 minutes.

Per serving: Calories: 699; Total Fat: 34g; Saturated Fat: 10g; Protein: 87g; Total Carbohydrates: 6g; Fiber: 1g; Sugar: 2g; Cholesterol: 408mg

OVEN-BAKED CHICKEN FINGERS

SERVES: 4   **PREP TIME:** 15 minutes   **COOK TIME:** 30 minutes

You love chicken fingers. There's no shame in that. You're a grown-ass man, you can like whatever you want. But if you are going to eat chicken fingers, why not eat the best ones you can? You can make these in large batches, cook them, and freeze them. Then you just have to reheat 'em and eat 'em.

¾ cup all-purpose flour

1 teaspoon salt

¼ teaspoon freshly ground black pepper

4 large eggs

1 cup fine dried bread crumbs

2 tablespoons poultry seasoning

¼ cup olive oil

2 boneless, skinless chicken breasts, sliced into strips

1. Preheat the oven to 400°F.

2. Set up a dredging station: In a small bowl, put the flour and season with the salt and pepper. In a second bowl, lightly beat the eggs. Combine the bread crumbs and poultry seasoning in a third bowl.

3. Spread the olive oil out onto a sheet pan.

4. Dip the chicken breast strips, one piece at a time, into the flour, then the egg, then the bread crumbs. Put the breaded chicken on a plate until all the pieces are coated.

5. Arrange the coated chicken on the sheet pan and cook for 15 minutes. Flip the fingers and bake for another 15 minutes, or until they're cooked through (165°F on a meat thermometer). Serve.

 FLAVOR BOOST: Serve the fingers with your favorite dipping sauce.

Per serving: Calories: 451; Total Fat: 22g; Saturated Fat: 4g; Protein: 24g; Total Carbohydrates: 39g; Fiber: 2g; Sugar: 2g; Cholesterol: 204mg

CLASSIC CARBONARA

SERVES: 1   **PREP TIME:** 5 minutes   **COOK TIME:** 10 minutes

Carbonara is an amazingly simple pasta dish that a lot of people get wrong. It might be the simplicity of the dish that confuses them. How can something so good be so simple? This carbonara is about as classic as you're going to get, with one exception. Typically a carbonara is made with guanciale, which is salt-cured pig cheek (it's better than it sounds), but since you probably aren't going to be able to find guanciale, this uses the more readily available pancetta.

Salt

2 ounces dried spaghetti

½ cup diced pancetta

3 large egg yolks

**¼ cup grated Parmesan cheese, plus
  1 tablespoon**

⅛ teaspoon freshly ground black pepper

1. Bring a medium pot of salted water to a boil. Add the pasta and cook according to package directions.

2. Meanwhile, warm a medium skillet over medium heat. Add the pancetta and cook 4 to 5 minutes, until crispy. Hold the pancetta and the rendered fat in the pan.

3. In a medium bowl, whisk together the egg yolks, ¼ cup of Parmesan, and the pepper. Whisk 2 tablespoons of the water from the pasta pot into the egg yolk mixture.

4. Drain the pasta and immediately add it to the bowl with the egg yolks. As soon as the pasta goes in the bowl, stir it with a set of tongs until the sauce is creamy. Add the pancetta along with 1 teaspoon of fat from the pan and continue to stir for another minute.

5. Taste the pasta and season with salt, if needed. Put the pasta in a serving bowl and top with the remaining 1 tablespoon of Parmesan.

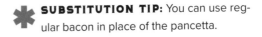 **SUBSTITUTION TIP:** You can use regular bacon in place of the pancetta.

Per serving: Calories: 621; Total Fat: 31g; Saturated Fat: 13g; Protein: 36g; Total Carbohydrates: 49g; Fiber: 2g; Sugar: 2g; Cholesterol: 502mg

CHICKEN PARMESAN

SERVES: 2   **PREP TIME:** 10 minutes   **COOK TIME:** 20 minutes

Chicken Parm is one of those things that just about everyone loves. It is breaded chicken that is smothered in marinara sauce, topped with cheese, and baked. The recipe below uses the chicken finger and marinara recipes from this book, but you can just as easily make this with store-bought chicken fingers and marinara sauce.

---

8 Oven-Baked Chicken Fingers (page 102)

**2 cups marinara sauce, homemade
   (page 150) or store-bought, divided**

**4 tablespoons grated Parmesan
   cheese, divided**

¼ cup shredded mozzarella cheese

Salt

4 ounces dried spaghetti

Freshly ground black pepper

---

1. Preheat the oven to 375°F.

2. Put the cooked chicken fingers in a small baking dish. Spoon 1 cup of marinara sauce over the chicken and cover with 2 tablespoons of Parmesan and all the mozzarella. Cover the pan with aluminum foil and bake in the oven for 20 minutes.

3. Bring a large pot of salted water to a boil and cook the pasta according to package directions.

4. Drain the pasta into a colander and let sit for a few minutes. Meanwhile, add the remaining 1 cup marinara sauce to the pasta pot, return the pot to the heat, and heat the sauce until it starts to bubble. As soon as the sauce is bubbling hot, remove the pot from the heat, add the pasta, and stir to coat it in the sauce.

5. Divide the pasta between two bowls and top with the chicken and remaining 2 tablespoons Parmesan. Season with salt and pepper, and serve.

Per serving: Calories: 949; Total Fat: 44g; Saturated Fat: 10g; Protein: 40g; Total Carbohydrates: 97g; Fiber: 6g; Sugar: 13g; Cholesterol: 227mg

SAUSAGE AND PEPPER PASTA SKILLET

SERVES: 2   **PREP TIME:** 10 minutes   **COOK TIME:** 20 minutes

There aren't many pasta dishes out there that can beat this sausage and pepper pasta skillet, so don't even try to find one. The bell pepper adds a little sweetness while the sausages provide a bit of spice and the bulk of the flavor. Top it all with gooey, melty mozzarella cheese and you have yourself a real winner.

Salt
4 ounces penne pasta
1 teaspoon olive oil
2 Italian sausages
1 red bell pepper, sliced
**1 cup marinara sauce, homemade (page 150)
  or store-bought**
¼ cup water
¾ cup shredded mozzarella cheese
Salt
Freshly ground black pepper

1. Position a rack in the center of the oven and turn the broiler to high.

2. Bring a large pot of salted water to a boil and cook the pasta according to package directions.

3. Meanwhile, warm a broilerproof medium skillet over medium heat. Add the olive oil and the sausages. Cook the sausages for about 3 minutes per side, or until browned.

4. Take the sausages out of the pan and set aside. Add the bell pepper into the pan and sauté for 3 minutes.

5. Slice the sausages into ¼-inch-thick pieces and return them to the pan along with the marinara and water. Reduce the heat to a simmer and cook the sauce for 5 minutes.

6. Drain the pasta, add to the skillet, and toss with the sauce. Cover with the mozzarella and put under the broiler for 1 to 2 minutes, until the cheese is melted and browned. Watch the pasta closely, as it can burn quickly. Season with salt and pepper, and serve.

❋ **FLAVOR BOOST:** Other ingredients like onion, garlic, green bell pepper, and spinach can be added to the pasta to bulk it up a bit.

Per serving: Calories: 814; Total Fat: 48g; Saturated Fat: 16g; Protein: 33g; Total Carbohydrates: 61g; Fiber: 5g; Sugar: 15g; Cholesterol: 99mg

PAN-SEARED STEAK WITH WHISKEY SAUCE

SERVES: 2   **PREP TIME:** 5 minutes, plus 5 minutes to rest   **COOK TIME:** 20 minutes

You know how people try to convince you to eat something by saying it will put hair on your chest? Well, this meal is so manly, just cooking it will put hair on your chest. You may be sprouting some right now just reading this.

2 sirloin steaks (4 to 5 ounces each)
Salt
Freshly ground black pepper
1 tablespoon olive oil
¼ cup whiskey
½ cup beef stock
2 tablespoons heavy cream
1 teaspoon Dijon mustard

1. Warm a medium skillet over medium-high heat. Season the steaks with salt and pepper. Add the oil and steaks to the pan and cook for 4 minutes per side. Take the steaks out of the pan and set aside to rest for 5 minutes.

2. Drain the fat out of the pan and pour in the whiskey. Cook the whiskey for about 30 seconds to cook off the alcohol. Add the beef stock, increase the heat to high, and bring to a boil. Boil the stock for about 3 minutes, or until reduced by half. Add the cream and cook for another 2 minutes.

3. Remove from the heat and stir in the mustard. Taste the sauce and season with salt and pepper as needed.

4. Pour any juices that have accumulated around the steaks into the sauce, stir, then pour the sauce over the steaks and serve.

Per serving: Calories: 420; Total Fat: 28g; Saturated Fat: 10g; Protein: 23g; Total Carbohydrates: 1g; Fiber: <1g; Sugar: 1g; Cholesterol: 107mg

PULLED PORK

SERVES: 8   **PREP TIME:** 5 minutes, plus 20 minutes to rest   **COOK TIME:** 3 hours

Pulled pork is good on sandwiches, tacos, tostadas, pasta, perogies, spoons, forks, and just about anything else. Seriously, try to think of something that pulled pork wouldn't be good on. Bet you can't.

---

1 teaspoon onion powder

1 teaspoon garlic powder

1 teaspoon smoked paprika

2 cups barbecue sauce, homemade (page 152) or store-bought

1 (5- to 6-pound) boneless pork shoulder

---

1. Preheat the oven to 325°F.

2. In a small bowl, combine the onion powder, garlic powder, smoked paprika, and barbecue sauce.

3. Rub half the mixture on the pork and set the rest of it aside. Put the pork in a roasting pan, cover tightly with aluminum foil, and put in the oven for 3 hours.

4. Take the pork out of the oven and test its doneness by poking it with a fork. If the meat easily comes apart, it's ready. If not, cover it back up and return it to the oven for another 30 minutes, then test it again.

5. When the pork is ready, take it out of the oven and let it rest for 20 minutes. Then pull it apart using two forks, mix in the reserved sauce, and serve.

Per serving: Calories: 580; Total Fat: 35g; Saturated Fat: 12g; Protein: 50g; Total Carbohydrates: 14g; Fiber: <1g; Sugar: 11g; Cholesterol: 176mg

SWEET AND STICKY PORK CHOPS

SERVES: 2 **PREP TIME:** 5 minutes **COOK TIME:** 20 minutes

These babies are delicious, and they make great leftovers. You can cut them into small pieces and add them to noodles, fried rice, salads, or all kinds of other things.

½ cup barbecue sauce, homemade (page 152) or store-bought

1 tablespoon light brown sugar

½ teaspoon paprika

¼ teaspoon cayenne pepper

¼ teaspoon salt

⅛ teaspoon freshly ground black pepper

4 bone-in pork loin chops

1. Preheat the oven to 400°F.

2. In a small bowl, mix together the barbecue sauce, brown sugar, paprika, cayenne, salt, and black pepper.

3. Pat the pork chops dry with a paper towel, brush with half the sauce, and place them in a roasting pan with a rack.

4. Roast the pork chops for 10 minutes. Flip them, brush them with the remaining sauce, and roast for another 10 minutes, or until the pork chops are cooked through (165°F).

Per serving: Calories: 746; Total Fat: 36g; Saturated Fat: 12g; Protein: 83g; Total Carbohydrates: 18g; Fiber: 1g; Sugar: 15g; Cholesterol: 275mg

CRISPY PORK TOSTADAS

SERVES: 2 **PREP TIME:** 5 minutes **COOK TIME:** 20 minutes

Tostadas are like big, round tortilla chips. You can find them at most grocery stores, and they make great flat, crispy tacos. If you've never tried them before, you may become slightly addicted to them. It's a real problem.

---

1 cup water

1 cup cubed (½-inch) pork shoulder (pork belly will also work)

¼ teaspoon salt

½ cup refried beans, homemade (page 71) or store-bought

4 tostadas

¼ cup diced tomatoes

¼ cup guacamole, homemade (page 48) or store-bought

---

1. In a medium pot, combine the water, pork, and salt and bring to a boil over medium heat. Reduce the heat to low and simmer uncovered until all of the water has evaporated. Continue to cook the pork, stirring every 2 to 3 minutes, until it's browned and crispy on all sides.

2. Meanwhile, heat the refried beans in the microwave on medium-high for about 1 minute, stop and stir them, then cook them for another minute or until hot.

3. Spread the beans on all 4 tostadas and top each with crispy pork and mozzarella. Put one tostada on top of the other to make two double-stack tostadas. Top each stack with guacamole.

❋ **SERVING TIP:** If dairy isn't an issue, sour cream makes for a great topper for these tostadas. If desired, simply drizzle the sour cream atop the tostadas after assembly and prior to serving.

Per serving: Calories: 482; Total Fat: 38g; Saturated Fat: 14g; Protein: 11g; Total Carbohydrates: 26g; Fiber: 5g; Sugar: 1g; Cholesterol: 41mg

CLASSIC ROAST CHICKEN

SERVES: 4 **PREP TIME:** 5 minutes, plus 20 minutes to rest
COOK TIME: 1 hour 30 minutes

Every person should know how to roast a chicken. It's not hard, it just takes time—even though most of that time you don't have to do anything. Plus, at the end you get a delicious roasted chicken.

---

1 whole chicken (5 pounds), giblets removed

2 tablespoons olive oil

2 teaspoons poultry seasoning

1 teaspoon paprika

1 teaspoon salt

½ teaspoon freshly ground black pepper

---

1. Preheat the oven to 375°F.

2. Pat the chicken dry inside and out with a paper towel. Rub the chicken all over with the olive oil.

3. In a small bowl, mix together the poultry seasoning, paprika, salt, and pepper.

4. Rub the spice blend all over the chicken, then place the chicken in a roasting pan with a rack, breast-side up.

5. Roast the chicken for 1 hour 30 minutes, or until a thermometer poked into the thickest part of the thigh and breast reaches a temperature of 170°F.

6. Remove the chicken from the oven and let it rest for at least 20 minutes before slicing into it.

Per serving: Calories: 422; Total Fat: 28g; Saturated Fat: 7g; Protein: 41g; Total Carbohydrates: 1g; Fiber: <1g; Sugar: <1g; Cholesterol: 132mg

LEMON AND CHILE CHICKEN LEGS

SERVES: 4 **PREP TIME:** 10 minutes, plus 1 hour to marinate **COOK TIME:** 40 minutes

Chicken with lemon and chile is a delicious combination. It also looks beautiful and it's super easy to make. Serve it with rice, roasted potatoes, or salad. Pull any leftover chicken off the bones and add it to salads for lunch.

4 skin-on chicken leg quarters (drumstick and thigh)

Grated zest and juice of 1 lemon

½ teaspoon red pepper flakes

Leaves from 8 to 10 sprigs thyme

4 garlic cloves, sliced

½ teaspoon salt

⅛ teaspoon freshly ground black pepper

2 tablespoons olive oil

1. Put the chicken in a large bowl and sprinkle with the lemon zest, lemon juice, pepper flakes, thyme, garlic, salt, pepper, and olive oil. Massage the herbs and spices into the chicken, cover the bowl, and refrigerate for 1 hour.

2. Preheat the oven to 400°F. Line a sheet pan with parchment paper.

3. Lay the chicken on the lined sheet pan and roast for 40 minutes, or until a thermometer inserted into the thickest part of the thigh reaches a temperature of 165°F.

SUBSTITUTION TIP: You can substitute 1 teaspoon dried thyme leaves or ½ teaspoon ground thyme for the fresh thyme.

Per serving: Calories: 803; Total Fat: 62g; Saturated Fat: 16g; Protein: 57g; Total Carbohydrates: 2g; Fiber: <1g; Sugar: <1g; Cholesterol: 320mg

SKILLET FRIED CHICKEN

SERVES: 2 **PREP TIME:** 10 minutes, plus 2 hours to marinate, 20 minutes to sit, and 5 minutes to rest **COOK TIME:** 15 minutes

There are two secrets to great fried chicken: using buttermilk, and letting the chicken sit in the flour for 20 minutes. The buttermilk keeps the chicken tender and adds a bit of flavor. Letting the chicken sit in the flour for 20 minutes dries the surface of the chicken out a little bit and creates a crust that gets super crispy when fried. The more you know!

2 boneless, skinless chicken breasts

¼ cup buttermilk

½ cup all-purpose flour

1 tablespoon poultry seasoning

½ teaspoon salt

¼ teaspoon freshly ground black pepper

1 cup canola oil

1. Lay the chicken breasts flat on your cutting board. Slice each chicken breast through the middle horizontally to create 2 thinner cutlets (for a total of 4 cutlets).

2. Put the chicken in a container, coat in the buttermilk, cover with plastic wrap and refrigerate for 2 hours.

3. In a medium bowl, mix the flour, poultry seasoning, salt, and pepper.

4. Take the chicken out of the buttermilk and let any excess drip off the breasts. Put the chicken in the flour mixture and toss to coat. Let the chicken sit in the flour for 20 minutes.

5. In a large skillet, heat the oil over medium heat until it reaches 360°F.

6. Put the chicken in the oil and cook for 6 minutes. Flip and cook for another 6 to 7 minutes, until the internal temperature of the chicken reaches 165°F.

7. Set the chicken on a wire rack and let it rest for 5 minutes before serving.

✳ **FLAVOR BOOST:** For a bit of a kick, add ¼ teaspoon cayenne pepper to the flour and/or a few teaspoons of hot sauce to the buttermilk.

Per serving: Calories: 510; Total Fat: 32g; Saturated Fat: 3g; Protein: 29g; Total Carbohydrates: 27g; Fiber: 1g; Sugar: 2g; Cholesterol: 83mg

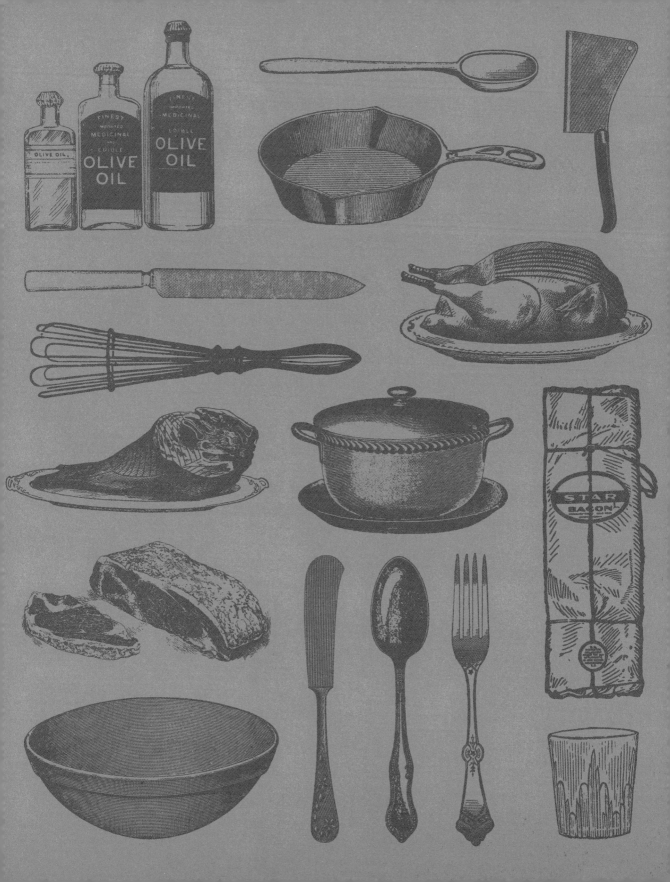

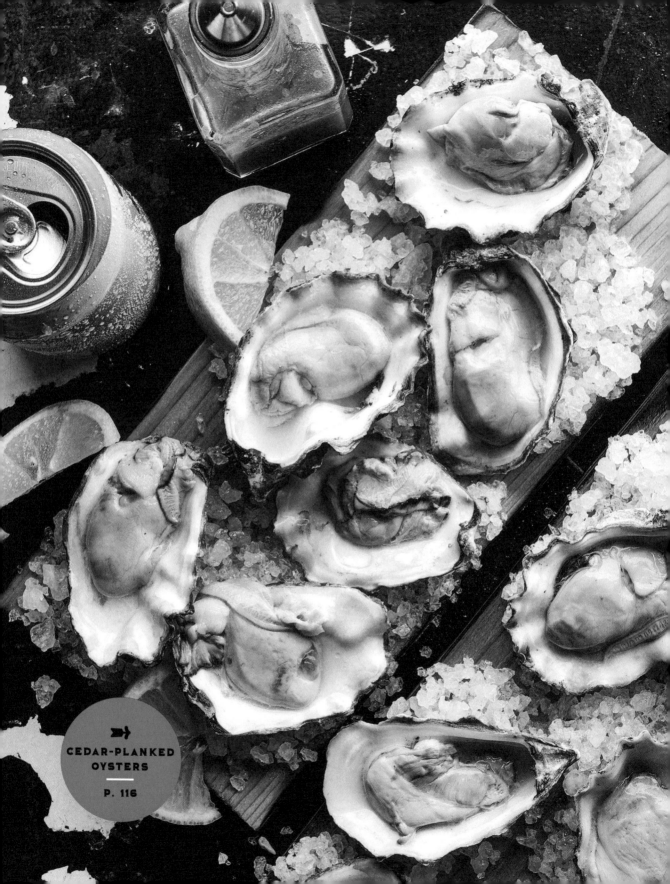

CEDAR-PLANKED
OYSTERS
—
P. 116

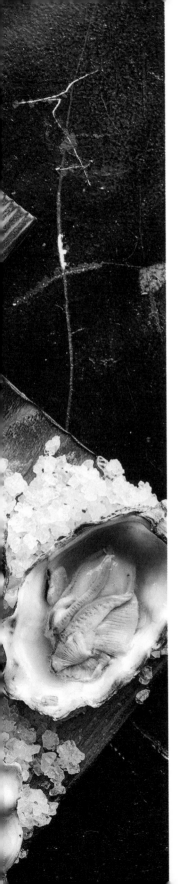

—8—
STRAPPING SEAFOOD

CEDAR-PLANKED OYSTERS

SERVES: 2   **PREP TIME:** 15 minutes, plus 1 hour to soak   **COOK TIME:** 15 minutes

It's hot. You're sitting on a patio overlooking the ocean with your best buds, sipping on an ice-cold beer. You feel a bit hungry. You spot the grill off in the corner and immediately get an idea. You grab your favorite axe and locate the best-looking cedar tree anyone has ever seen. Within minutes, using nothing but your wits and good looks, you've carved a perfectly flat plank of wood. You set the plank aside, jump in the nearby ocean, and 10 minutes later you surface with a bucket of fresh oysters. You light the grill, throw the piece of cedar (or two, depending on the size) on the grates, and top it with the oysters. Everyone cheers your name as the smoke from the plank cooks and flavors the oysters. Just another day in paradise.

1. Soak the cedar plank(s) in water for 1 hour before use.

2. Heat a gas grill to 400°F.

3. Mix the salt and water and divide the mixture into 12 even mounds on the soaked cedar plank, about 2 inches apart.

4. Open an oyster shell using an oyster knife, loosen the oyster from the bottom shell, and place the shell on one mound of salt. Repeat this process until all of the oysters are open.

5. Carefully put the cedar plank(s) on the grill, turn your burners to medium-low, and close the grill. Bake the oysters for 10 to 12 minutes.

6. Remove the plank(s) from the grill, squeeze the lemon over the oysters, and add a few drops of hot sauce to each one.

7. Serve with a cold beer (optional).

1 cedar plank (or 2 smaller ones)

1 cup coarse salt

¼ cup water

12 oysters

1 lemon, cut into wedges

Hot sauce

Per serving: Calories: 220; Total Fat: 6g; Saturated Fat: 1g; Protein: 26g; Total Carbohydrates: 14g; Fiber: 0g; Sugar: 0g; Cholesterol: 136mg

SCALLOP CEVICHE

SERVES: 2   **PREP TIME:** 5 minutes, plus 10 minutes to sit

Imagine you're sitting on a beach, the warm sand wrapped around your toes. You've been there all day and are starting to get hungry. A beach vendor walks buy and offers you a snack. You accept, take a bite, and are instantly hit with the taste of summer, ocean, and sunshine. That was scallop ceviche—and with the recipe below, you can now have that feeling whenever you want. Enjoy the ceviche on its own or with tortilla chips. Yeah, you're welcome.

1 pound sea scallops, diced

1 sweet orange, cut into segments

1 tablespoon fresh lime juice

1 tablespoon minced jalapeño pepper

3 tablespoons minced red onion

½ teaspoon salt

⅛ teaspoon freshly ground black pepper

2 teaspoons olive oil

1. In a medium nonmetallic bowl, combine the scallops, orange segments, lime juice, jalapeño, red onion, salt, pepper, and olive oil. Stir the ingredients well and let sit for 10 minutes.

2. Taste the mixture and season with a bit more salt and pepper, if needed.

3. Serve.

✳ **INGREDIENT TIP:** If you prefer a milder flavor, remove the seeds and white ribs from the jalapeño. Add a bit of fresh cilantro for a pop of summer flavor.

✳ **PREP TIP:** To segment the orange, peel it, then use a small sharp knife to cut the segments free from the membranes. This will give you cleaner, better-looking, and easier-to-eat pieces of orange than if you pulled the orange apart by hand and left the membranes on.

Per serving: Calories: 216; Total Fat: 6g; Saturated Fat: 1g; Protein: 29g; Total Carbohydrates: 13g; Fiber: 2g; Sugar: 7g; Cholesterol: 60mg

MISO SCALLOP SKEWERS

SERVES: 3　**PREP TIME:** 5 minutes, plus 1 hour to soak　**COOK TIME:** 5 minutes

Miso is a paste made of fermented soybeans that dates back to the fourth century BCE. Yeah, that's a long time. Miso is super salty, so a little goes a long way. Scallops are naturally sweet so something salty pairs with them well—that's why bacon and scallops is such a common pairing. In this recipe the miso takes the place of the bacon to create a delicious naturally sweet and salty scallop.

2 tablespoons mayonnaise

1 tablespoon miso

2 teaspoons honey

1 teaspoon sriracha

1 pound sea scallops (20/30)
  (see Ingredient Tip)

1. Soak six 6-inch bamboo skewers in water for 1 hour.

2. Heat the grill to 450°F.

3. In a small bowl, stir together the mayonnaise, miso, honey, and sriracha.

4. Thread the scallops onto the skewers and brush the scallops with the miso glaze. Put the skewers on the grill and cook for 2 minutes. Flip the scallops and brush with more of the glaze and cook for another 2 minutes, then flip and brush again.

5. The scallops are cooked when they are firm to the touch but not rubbery. It is better to undercook scallops slightly than to overcook them.

✳ INGREDIENT TIP: Scallops and shrimp are often sold and labeled according to the number of them you would get in a pound. For example 20/30 sea scallops means that there are 20 to 30 scallops in a pound. Really large scallops are U10s, which means that there are 10 or fewer scallops in a pound.

Per serving: Calories: 181; Total Fat: 8g; Saturated Fat: 1g; Protein: 20g; Total Carbohydrates: 8g; Fiber: <1g; Sugar: 4g; Cholesterol: 44mg

TEQUILA LIME SHRIMP

SERVES: 2　**PREP TIME:** 5 minutes　**COOK TIME:** 10 minutes

These shrimp are a great snack, party hors d'oeuvre, or addition to a burrito, taco, wrap, or salad. You can even serve them over rice to make them a meal. Finish the shrimp with some chopped fresh cilantro for a pop of color and flavor.

1 tablespoon olive oil

1 pound shrimp, peeled

½ teaspoon salt

½ teaspoon red pepper flakes

2 tablespoons tequila

Grated zest and juice of 1 lime

1 tablespoon salted butter

1. Warm a medium skillet over medium-high heat. Add the olive oil and shrimp to the pan, season with the salt and pepper flakes, and cook for 2 minutes per side.

2. Add the tequila to the pan and let it cook for 1 minute, or until it has mostly all evaporated.

3. Flip the shrimp, add the lime zest, lime juice, and butter. Remove from the heat and stir until the butter melts.

4. Put the shrimp on a plate and pour the sauce over them.

✳ **PREP TIP:** Shrimp take a lot less time to cook than most people think. As soon as they turn pink, they're good to go. When they're overcooked, they're rubbery and bland. Perfectly cooked shrimp are tender and flavorful.

Per serving: Calories: 308; Total Fat: 15g; Saturated Fat: 5g; Protein: 30g; Total Carbohydrates: 4g; Fiber: <1g; Sugar: <1g; Cholesterol: 305mg

FISH TACOS

SERVES: 2 **PREP TIME:** 5 minutes **COOK TIME:** 5 minutes

There's a pretty good chance that you love tacos. Everyone does, right? Well, get ready for that healthy love of tacos to become an unhealthy obsession, because these fish tacos are addictive as all hell.

---

1 pound halibut, cut into 1-inch-wide strips

1 tablespoon Cajun seasoning

¼ teaspoon salt

1 tablespoon olive oil

6 (4-inch) corn tortillas

¼ cup black bean salsa, homemade (page 49) or store-bought

¼ cup diced pineapple

---

1. Warm a nonstick skillet over medium-high heat. Season the halibut strips with the Cajun seasoning and salt. Add the olive oil and halibut strips to the pan and cook for 2 to 3 minutes per side.

2. Warm the tortillas according to the package directions.

3. Put the fish on the warmed tortillas, top with salsa and pineapple, and serve.

✳ **FLAVOR BOOST:** Garnish the tacos with fresh jalapeño, cilantro, and a squeeze of fresh lime for an extra pop of flavor.

Per serving: Calories: 400; Total Fat: 11g; Saturated Fat: 2g; Protein: 45g; Total Carbohydrates: 25g; Fiber: 5g; Sugar: 5g; Cholesterol: 111mg

OVEN-BAKED FISH FINGERS

MAKES: 24 fish fingers   **PREP TIME:** 15 minutes   **COOK TIME:** 15 minutes

These fish fingers are quick, easy, and delicious. They are the perfect food for the kid in you. Serve them with some crinkle-cut fries and a pile of ketchup in front of the TV for the full childhood experience.

1 cup all-purpose flour

½ teaspoon salt

¼ teaspoon freshly ground black pepper

3 large eggs, beaten

1 cup fine dried bread crumbs

¼ cup olive oil

2 pounds haddock, cut into 24 finger-width strips

1. Preheat the oven to 425°F.

2. Set up a dredging station in three shallow bowls: In one, season the flour with the salt and pepper. Place the eggs in a second bowl and the bread crumbs in a third.

3. Spread the olive oil in an even layer on a sheet pan.

4. Dip each piece of haddock first in the seasoned flour, then the egg, then the bread crumbs. Put the coated haddock on a plate as you work.

5. Arrange the breaded fish fingers on the baking sheet with a little space between them. Bake the fingers in the oven for 7 minutes. Flip and bake for another 7 minutes, or until golden brown on both sides.

PREP TIP: When breading the haddock, try to use one hand for the flour and bread crumbs and one hand to pick up the fish and dip it in the egg wash. This is called "wet hand dry hand" and it will keep you from breading your fingers.

STORAGE TIP: Once cooked, the fish fingers can be frozen for up to 4 months. They can be reheated from frozen in a 400°F oven for about 12 minutes per side.

Per serving (4 fish fingers): Calories: 304; Total Fat: 10g; Saturated Fat: 1.5g; Protein: 30g; Total Carbohydrates: 22g; Fiber: 1g; Sugar: 1g; Cholesterol: 148mg

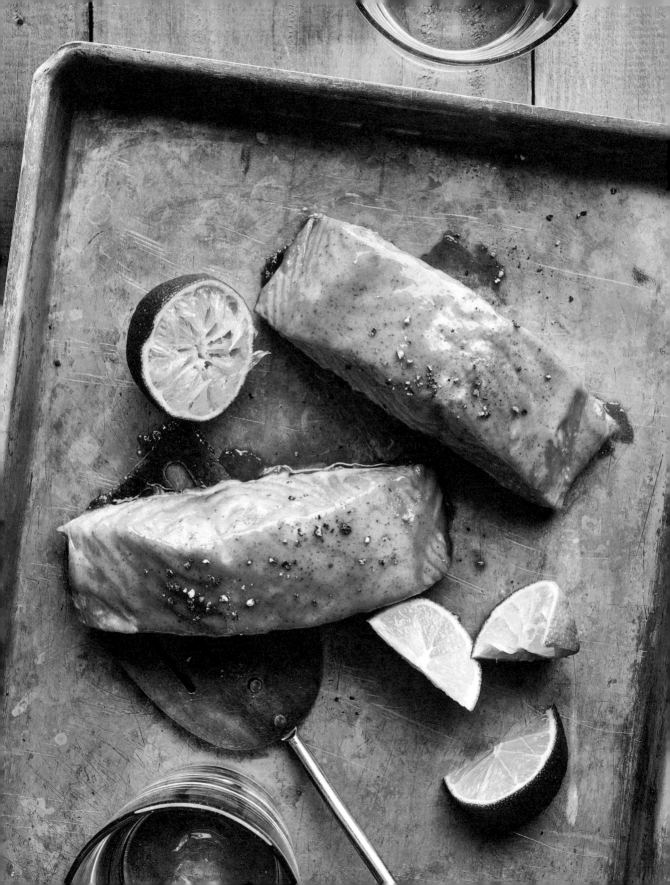

MAPLE-PEPPER SALMON

SERVES: 2 **PREP TIME:** 5 minutes, plus 1 hour to marinate **COOK TIME:** 25 minutes

Salmon—if it's good enough for a grizzly bear, it's good enough for you. Luckily, unlike grizzly bears, you don't have to catch a fish and rip it apart with your bare hands. I mean you can, all the power to you. But, even better than that, you can cook the salmon and load it up with flavor. Serve the salmon with Cauliflower Rice (page 93).

¼ **cup maple syrup**

1 teaspoon freshly ground black pepper

1 **tablespoon Dijon mustard**

2 **scallions, sliced**

2 **salmon fillets (6 ounces each)**

1. In a medium bowl, whisk together the maple syrup, pepper, Dijon mustard, and scallions. Put the salmon in a large zip-top bag and pour the maple mixture over it. Pinch as much air out of the bag as you can, seal it, roll the salmon around to coat it in the sauce, and refrigerate for 1 hour to marinate.

2. When the salmon has been marinating for 40 minutes, preheat the oven to 350°F.

3. Take the salmon out of the marinade and use your fingers to wipe away any excess. Arrange the salmon on a broiler pan and bake for 15 to 20 minutes. Check that the salmon is cooked by using a fork to gently open the fish at its thickest point. If the center of the salmon is translucent, cook it for another 4 to 5 minutes.

Per serving: Calories: 356; Total Fat: 11g; Saturated Fat: 2g; Protein: 34g; Total Carbohydrates: 28g; Fiber: 1g; Sugar: 24g; Cholesterol: 94mg

SRIRACHA-LIME SALMON

SERVES: 2   **PREP TIME:** 5 minutes   **COOK TIME:** 15 minutes

There's nothing that you can't put sriracha-lime mayonnaise on. Yeah, it works well on salmon, but you can also use it on oysters, chicken salad, a roast beef sandwich, tacos, or just about anything else. Having said that, salmon is a great choice when you want to eat healthy, but like, not that healthy. You know?

---

2 tablespoons mayonnaise

1 tablespoon sriracha

1 tablespoon fresh lime juice

1 teaspoon honey

2 salmon fillets (6 ounces each)

Oil, for the pan

---

1. Preheat the oven to 400°F.

2. In a medium bowl, whisk together the mayonnaise, sriracha, lime juice, and honey.

3. Put the salmon on a lightly oiled broiler pan. Brush the salmon with the sriracha-lime mayonnaise.

4. Put the salmon in the oven and bake for 12 to 15 minutes, until the fish is just cooked.

Per serving: Calories: 348; Total Fat: 21g; Saturated Fat: 3g; Protein: 34g; Total Carbohydrates: 4g; Fiber: 0g; Sugar: 3g; Cholesterol: 99mg

SEAFOOD PASTA

SERVES: 2   **PREP TIME:** 5 minutes   **COOK TIME:** 15 minutes

One of the great things about seafood pasta is that you can use just about any seafood you want. This recipe uses clams, shrimp, and haddock, but it could easily be scallops, mussels, and salmon. Use whatever seafood you like. If you want something to cook to impress your mom and show her that you're doing all right, this is the thing.

1 (5-ounce) can clams

¼ teaspoon salt, plus more to season water

4 ounces dried spaghetti

1 tablespoon olive oil

4 ounces shrimp, peeled

4 ounces haddock, cut into 1-inch pieces

1 cup marinara sauce, homemade (page 150) or store-bought

¼ teaspoon freshly ground black pepper

1. Set a sieve over a small bowl and dump the can of clams in. Set the drained clams and clam liquid aside.

2. Bring a large pot of salted water to a boil over high heat. Add the pasta and cook according to the package directions.

3. Meanwhile, warm a large skillet over medium-high heat. Add the olive oil and shrimp and cook for 1 minute per side. Add the juice from the clams and cook until the liquid has reduced by half its volume, about 4 to 5 minutes.

4. Add the haddock and marinara sauce to the skillet, reduce the heat to medium, and cook for 4 to 5 minutes, until the sauce is hot and the haddock is cooked. Season the sauce with ¼ teaspoon salt and the pepper.

5. Drain the pasta and add it to the sauce along with the clams. Toss the pasta to coat in the sauce and serve.

✱ **FLAVOR BOOST:** Finish the pasta with some chopped fresh parsley, a pinch of red pepper flakes, and a spoonful of garlic butter to elevate the flavor.

Per serving: Calories: 601; Total Fat: 24g; Saturated Fat: 3g; Protein: 37g; Total Carbohydrates: 58g; Fiber: 4g; Sugar: 11g; Cholesterol: 123mg

BACON AND CLAM CHOWDER

SERVES: 4   **PREP TIME:** 5 minutes   **COOK TIME:** 30 minutes

Whether you're the type of man who's out chopping wood all day, or the type who's out fishing in the rough, salty spray of the ocean—or any other kind of man, really—clam chowder (or chow-da) is going to fill you up and make you feel good. It tastes just as good on a cold winter evening as it does on a sunny summer afternoon. Essentially, it's good any time of day or year.

1 (5-ounce) can clams

4 slices bacon, cut into 1-inch pieces

½ cup diced onion

1 cup small-diced peeled potatoes

3 cups heavy cream

½ teaspoon salt

¼ teaspoon freshly ground black pepper

1. Set a sieve over a small bowl and dump the can of clams in. Set the drained clams and clam liquid aside.

2. Put the bacon in a medium pot and set the pot over medium heat. Cook for 7 to 8 minutes, until it's browned and crispy.

3. Drain off all but 1 tablespoon of bacon fat from the pot. Add the onion and potatoes and cook for 3 minutes.

4. Add the clam liquid and cook for 4 minutes, or until the liquid has almost completely evaporated.

5. Add the cream and cook until hot. Reduce the heat to low and simmer the chowder for about 10 minutes, or until the potatoes are firm-tender.

6. Stir in the clams and let them heat through for about 1 minute. Season the chowder with the salt and pepper and serve.

Per serving: Calories: 712; Total Fat: 68g; Saturated Fat: 42g; Protein: 14 g; Total Carbohydrates: 15g; Fiber: 1g; Sugar: 7g; Cholesterol: 220mg

FISH IN PAPER

SERVES: 2   **PREP TIME:** 5 minutes   **COOK TIME:** 20 minutes

Cooking fish in paper does two things. Number one, it traps all the steam and flavor in a tight little package, making the fish tender and flavorful. Number two, it cuts down on dishes. In other words, a win-win.

1 teaspoon olive oil

2 (6-ounce) cod fillets

1 cup baby spinach

¼ teaspoon red pepper flakes

¼ cup white wine

½ cup marinara sauce, homemade (page 150) or store-bought

½ teaspoon salt

¼ teaspoon freshly ground black pepper

1. Preheat the oven to 375°F.

2. Warm a nonstick medium skillet over medium-high heat. Add the olive oil and fish and sear for about 2 minutes, or until browned on one side. Flip the fish and cook for another minute. Take the fish out of the pan and place each fillet on ½ of a 12-by-12-inch piece of parchment paper.

3. Add the spinach and pepper flakes to the skillet and cook for 1 minute, then add the wine and cook for another 2 minutes. Add the marinara and season with salt and pepper. Once the sauce is hot, take the pan off the heat.

4. Spoon the sauce over the fish. Fold the open side of the parchment over the fish (like closing a book) and fold and crimp all along the edges of the parchment to seal the packet. Put the fish packages on a baking sheet and bake in the oven for 12 minutes.

 PREP TIP: You can use foil instead of parchment paper.

Per serving: Calories: 272; Total Fat: 11g; Saturated Fat: 2g; Protein: 31g; Total Carbohydrates: 8g; Fiber: 1g; Sugar: 5g; Cholesterol: 88mg

HALIBUT CACCIATORE

SERVES: 2   **PREP TIME:** 5 minutes   **COOK TIME:** 15 minutes

Cacciatore is a dish traditionally made of chicken braised in tomato sauce with olives, herbs, and capers. This recipe switches the chicken for halibut, gets rid of the capers, and cuts down on the cooking time to fit it into your busy schedule.

1 teaspoon olive oil

2 halibut fillets (6 ounces each)

¼ cup white wine

½ cup marinara sauce, homemade (page 150) or store-bought

12 green olives

1 teaspoon chopped fresh thyme

¼ teaspoon salt

¼ teaspoon freshly ground black pepper

1. Warm a nonstick medium skillet over medium-high heat. Add the olive oil and the halibut and cook the fish on one side for 4 minutes, or until golden brown. Flip the fish, add the white wine, and cook for 2 minutes.

2. Add the marinara, olives, thyme, salt, and pepper. Cover, reduce the heat to low, and simmer for 5 to 7 minutes, until the fish is cooked through.

Per serving: Calories: 323; Total Fat: 15g; Saturated Fat: 2g; Protein: 33g; Total Carbohydrates: 8g; Fiber: 2g; Sugar: 5g; Cholesterol: 83mg

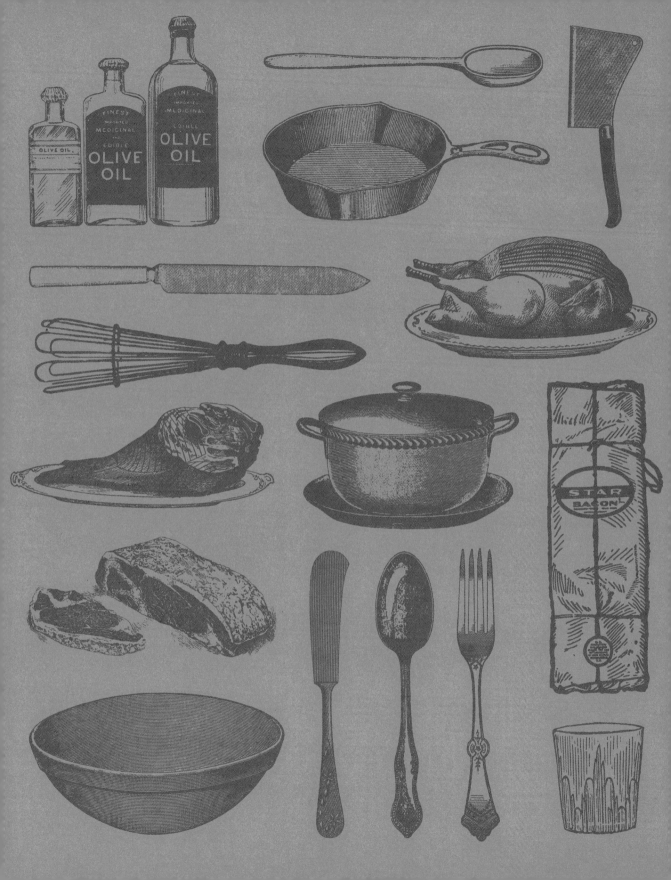

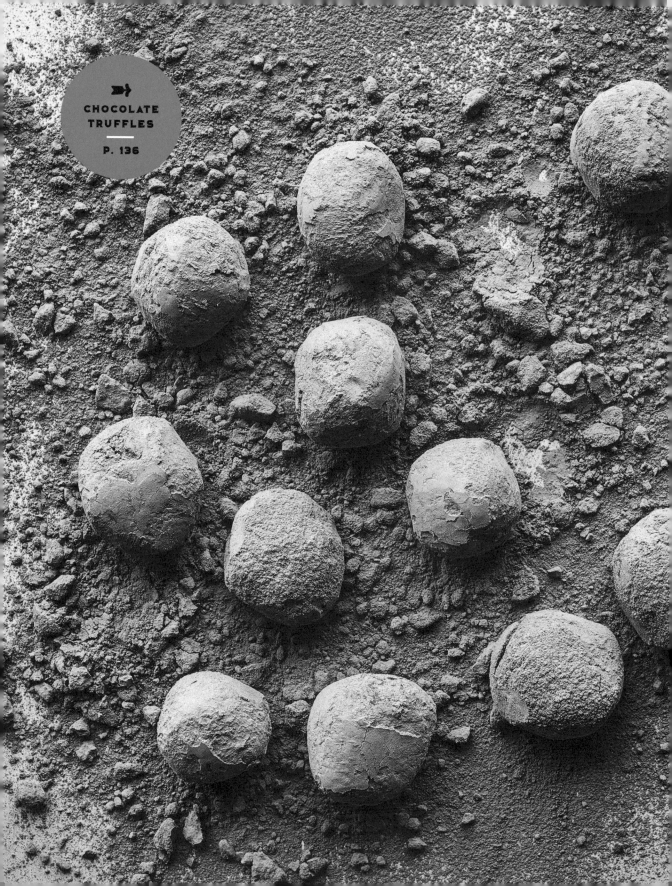

CHOCOLATE
TRUFFLES

P. 136

DECADENT DESSERTS AND BEVERAGES

POACHED PEARS

SERVES: 2   **PREP TIME:** 5 minutes, plus time to cool   **COOK TIME:** 25 minutes

Poached pears make a great dessert, but they're also delicious on salads with goat cheese and arugula. They even make a terrific garnish for a charcuterie or cheese board. You can do a lot with these little guys.

---

2 Bosc pears, cored and peeled

2 cups water

½ cinnamon stick

½ cup honey

¼ cup Bourbon Caramel Sauce (page 153)

2 scoops vanilla ice cream

---

1. In a medium pot, combine the pears, water, cinnamon stick, and honey. Bring to a boil over high heat, then turn the heat to low, cover, and simmer for 15 to 20 minutes, until the pears are tender.

2. Take the pears out of the liquid and let them cool.

3. Increase the heat under the pot to medium-high and cook until the liquid is as thick as pancake syrup, about 8 to 10 minutes. Discard the cinnamon stick and stir the caramel sauce into the reduced liquid.

4. Scoop the ice cream and place in a bowl beside a pear. Pour the caramel sauce over the pears and ice cream and serve.

✳ STORAGE TIP: If you want to make the pears ahead, poach them as directed and take out of the poaching liquid. Skip the step that says to boil the liquid until thick. Let the pear and cooking liquid cool separately, then pour the liquid over the pears and store in the refrigerator for up to 1 week.

Per serving: Calories: 823; Total Fat: 26g; Saturated Fat: 16g; Protein: 6g; Total Carbohydrates: 146g; Fiber: 7g; Sugar: 13g; Cholesterol: 92mg

APPLE GALETTE

SERVES: 8 **PREP TIME:** 10 minutes, plus 10 minutes to cool **COOK TIME:** 35 minutes

A galette is like a French free-form pie. Yeah, dude, you're fancy. Puff pastry creates a light and flaky crust and is easier than making pie crust from scratch. You may never want a classic apple pie again. To really kick this thing into high gear, finish it with a bit of the Bourbon Caramel Sauce (page 153).

6 cups Granny Smith apples, sliced and peeled

½ cup packed light brown sugar

2 tablespoons cornstarch

½ teaspoon ground cinnamon

¼ teaspoon salt

1 sheet frozen puff pastry, thawed

1. Position a rack in the center of the oven and preheat the oven to 400°F. Line a baking sheet with parchment paper.

2. In a large bowl, toss the sliced apples with the brown sugar, cornstarch, cinnamon, and salt.

3. Lay the puff pastry out on the lined baking sheet. Spread the apples in an even layer over the pastry, leaving a ½-inch border around the outside edge.

4. Fold the edges of the pastry up and over the apples to form the crust.

5. Bake the galette for 25 to 35 minutes, until the crust is browned and crisp. Let the galette cool for 10 minutes before cutting and serving.

✳ INGREDIENT TIP: If you want this to be dairy-free, seek out a puff pastry not made with butter.

Per serving: Calories: 186; Total Fat: 5g; Saturated Fat: 5g; Protein: 2g; Total Carbohydrates: 35g; Fiber: 4g; Sugar: 21g; Cholesterol: 0mg

PEACH GALETTE

SERVES: 8 **PREP TIME:** 10 minutes, plus 10 minutes to cool **COOK TIME:** 35 minutes

Peaches, puff pastry, honey, and ricotta cheese. As you will see, that's all you really need. Make this for a fancy dinner, a dinner party, or just when you deserve something delicious because you've been killing it lately.

---

1 cup ricotta cheese

¼ cup honey, plus 2 tablespoons

1 sheet frozen puff pastry, thawed

6 peaches, sliced

2 tablespoons cornstarch

---

1. Preheat the oven to 400°F. Line a baking sheet with parchment paper.

2. In a medium bowl, mix the ricotta with ¼ cup of honey.

3. Lay the puff pastry out on the lined baking sheet. Spread the ricotta/honey mixture out on the pastry, leaving a ½-inch border around the outside edge.

4. Toss the peaches with the cornstarch, then spread out on the ricotta. Fold the pastry, edge up over the peaches.

5. Drizzle the remaining 2 tablespoons of honey over the peaches. Bake for 25 to 35 minutes, until the pastry is golden brown.

6. Let the galette cool for 10 minutes before cutting and serving.

✱ SUBSTITUTION TIP: Swap out the ricotta cheese for 8 ounces cream cheese mixed with 2 tablespoons heavy cream.

Per serving: Calories: 217; Total Fat: 8g; Saturated Fat: 4g; Protein: 4g; Total Carbohydrates: 35g; Fiber: 2g; Sugar: 23g; Cholesterol: 15mg

NO-BAKE CHOCOLATE CHEESECAKE CUPS

SERVES: 4 **PREP TIME:** 15 minutes, plus 1 hour to set

You know who loves cheesecake? Everyone! Just because you're a dude doesn't mean you can't love something as delicious and amazing as a cheesecake. But here's the thing: Cheesecake is kind of a pain in the ass to make. Luckily, this recipe is super simple and gives you the taste of a great chocolate cheesecake without all the work. Get ready to impress that special lady in your life: your mom. Yes, your mom is going to be super impressed by this.

8 ounces cream cheese, at room temperature

½ cup heavy cream

¼ cup sugar

¼ cup unsweetened cocoa powder

1 cup chocolate cookie crumbs

1. In a bowl, with an electric mixer, beat the cream cheese until it is smooth. Add the heavy cream and sugar and beat until it is fully combined. Add the cocoa to the mix and beat on low until it is fully mixed in.

2. Grab four 16-ounce cups and put the cookie crumbs in the bottom of the cups. Top with the cheese mixture. Cover the cups with plastic wrap and refrigerate for 1 hour to set.

✳ INGREDIENT TIP: You can buy chocolate cookie crumbs in the baking aisle of the grocery store. Any leftover cookie crumbs can be used as a topping for ice cream or vanilla yogurt.

Per serving: Calories: 546; Total Fat: 39g; Saturated Fat: 21g; Protein: 8g; Total Carbohydrates: 48g; Fiber: 3g; Sugar: 32g; Cholesterol: 91mg

CHOCOLATE TRUFFLES

SERVES: 2   **PREP TIME:** 15 minutes, plus 4 hours to chill   **COOK TIME:** 5 minutes

Truffles are, like, super fancy. That means they must also be super hard to make, right? Nope. You won't believe how easy it is to make chocolate truffles. The trick is to not eat them all at once.

½ cup heavy cream
1 cup semisweet chocolate chips
1 tablespoon salted butter
1 tablespoon rum
¼ cup unsweetened cocoa powder

1. In a small pot, bring the cream to a boil. Put the chocolate in a heatproof medium bowl. Pour the hot cream over the chocolate and let it sit for 2 to 3 minutes. Whisk the chocolate until smooth.

2. Whisk in the butter. Then whisk in the rum.

3. Lay plastic wrap directly on the surface of the chocolate and put it in the fridge for at least 4 hours.

4. Take the chocolate out of the fridge. Spoon out a tablespoon-size ball of chocolate and roll it in the cocoa powder. Repeat the process until all the chocolate mix has been rolled in the cocoa.

 STORAGE TIP: Store the truffles in the fridge in an airtight container.

Per serving: Calories: 731; Total Fat: 56g; Saturated Fat: 34g; Protein: 8g; Total Carbohydrates: 66g; Fiber: 9g; Sugar: 52g; Cholesterol: 83mg

ORANGE TIRAMISU

SERVES: 4   **PREP TIME:** 15 minutes, plus 2 hours to chill

Tiramisu is a classic Italian dessert made of mascarpone cheese, ladyfinger cookies, and coffee. This version switches it up and flavors it with orange. Essentially, this tastes like an orange cream ice pop—and that's a very good thing.

1 cup heavy cream

1 cup sugar, divided

Grated zest and juice of 1 navel orange

1 cup mascarpone cheese

½ cup hot water

24 ladyfinger cookies

1. In a medium bowl, with an electric mixer, whip the cream and ½ cup of sugar together until the cream holds firm peaks.

2. In a separate bowl, mix together the orange zest, orange juice, and mascarpone. Fold the whipped cream into the mascarpone mixture.

3. In a small bowl, stir together the hot water and remaining ½ cup of sugar.

4. Grab four 16-ounce cups and put a spoonful of mascarpone mixture in the bottom of each.

5. Dip a ladyfinger in the sugar water and put it on top of the mascarpone mixture in the cup. You may have to break the cookies. Spoon more of the mascarpone mixture over the cookie. Repeat until all the cookies and the mascarpone mixture are used up, making sure the last layer in each cup is mascarpone mixture.

6. Cover the cups and refrigerate for at least 2 hours before serving.

✳ SUBSTITUTION TIP: You can use a different kind of sweet orange if you'd prefer, but try to get one that's about the size of a baseball. Otherwise, you may need to adjust the measurements.

Per serving: Calories: 838; Total Fat: 50g; Saturated Fat: 29g; Protein: 12g; Total Carbohydrates: 86g; Fiber: 1g; Sugar: 68g; Cholesterol: 249mg

CRÈME BRÛLÉE

SERVES: 4 **PREP TIME:** 15 minutes, plus 2 hours to chill **COOK TIME:** 45 minutes

Crème brûlée is such cool dessert. Chilled custard on the bottom, crispy caramelized sugar on top. You get to use a torch. What's cooler than fire? Nothing. Enjoy this, you beautiful bastard.

2 cups heavy cream
4 large eggs yolks
½ cup sugar, plus 4 tablespoons
1 teaspoon vanilla extract

1. Preheat the oven to 325°F.

2. In a medium pot, bring the cream to a boil. Remove from the heat and set aside.

3. In a heatproof medium bowl, whisk together the egg yolks and ½ cup of sugar until the yolks turn a pale yellow. Whisk the cream into the egg mixture, a few drops at a time to start. Slowly add the rest of the cream and whisk until all of the cream has been mixed into the eggs. Whisk in the vanilla.

4. Place a paper towel in the bottom of a roasting pan, then place four ramekins or ceramic mugs in the pan. Divide the egg mixture among the four 6-ounce ramekins, then fill the roasting pan with hot water until it reaches halfway up the sides of the ramekins.

5. Cover the roasting pan with foil and bake for 40 to 45 minutes, until the custard is set but still a little wobbly in the middle.

6. Take the ramekins out of the water, let cool slightly, then cover with plastic and refrigerate for 2 hours.

7. Evenly sprinkle the top of each cup of custard with 1 tablespoon of sugar and use a kitchen blowtorch to brûlé it just until the sugar is melted and browned.

Per serving: Calories: 600; Total Fat: 47g; Saturated Fat: 29g; Protein: 6g; Total Carbohydrates: 42g; Fiber: 0g; Sugar: 41g; Cholesterol: 293mg

ORANGE SODA POP

    VG

SERVES: 4   **PREP TIME:** 5 minutes, plus 1 hour to cool   **COOK TIME:** 15 minutes

Do you ever want to feel like a kid again? Well, now you can. Make this orange soda, curl up with a big bowl of popcorn, and throw on a movie. You'll feel like you're six years old in no time.

1 navel orange

½ cup sugar

1 cup water

2 teaspoons fresh lemon juice

4 cups sparkling water

1. Using a vegetable peeler, pull off strips of zest from the orange. Squeeze the orange juice and set aside.

2. In a medium pot, combine the sugar, tap water, and orange zest strips. Bring to a boil, reduce the heat to low, and simmer for 10 minutes. Remove from the heat and let cool completely.

3. Take the zest strips out of the syrup and stir in the orange juice and lemon juice.

4. Divide the syrup among four glasses. Top each with 1 cup of sparkling water and finish with lots of ice.

✱ FLAVOR BOOST: You can add some lemon and lime zest to make more of a citrus soda.

Per serving: Calories: 118; Total Fat: 0g; Saturated Fat: 0g; Protein: <1g; Total Carbohydrates: 30g; Fiber: 1g; Sugar: 29g; Cholesterol: 0mg

HOT CHOCOLATE

SERVES: 2 **PREP TIME:** 5 minutes **COOK TIME:** 10 minutes

It's a cold winter day, you've been out chopping trees in the forest. Not out of anger—it's your job. You've got a mighty chill that goes right through your bones. What are you to do? What could possibly warm you up after a long day of tree chopping? Hot Chocolate, that's what.

---

2 cups whole milk

¼ cup unsweetened cocoa powder

2 tablespoons sugar

¼ cup Irish cream

2 candy canes

---

1. In a medium pot, heat the milk over medium heat. Do not boil!

2. In a small bowl, combine the cocoa and sugar until evenly combined. Spoon 3 tablespoons of the mixture into each of two mugs. Add half Irish cream to each mug and stir to make paste.

3. Stir half the milk into each mug. Take the plastic off the candy canes, put one in each mug, and serve.

Per serving: Calories: 383; Total Fat: 14g; Saturated Fat: 8g; Protein: 11g; Total Carbohydrates: 52g; Fiber: 4g; Sugar: 41g; Cholesterol: 42mg

TACO JUICE

SERVES: 2 **PREP TIME:** 5 minutes

Do you love tacos but hate all the chewing? Who doesn't? Now you can have the wonderful flavor of a taco but in juice form. Okay, this doesn't taste exactly like a taco—would you even want it to? But it does taste delicious.

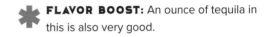

6 fresh cilantro leaves

¼ teaspoon chili powder

Grated zest and juice of 1 lime

1 cup orange-pineapple juice

1 cup sparkling water

1. Dividing evenly, put the cilantro, chili powder, lime zest, and lime juice in the bottom of two tall glasses and smash it a little bit with the end of a wooden spoon.

2. Stir in the orange-pineapple juice and fill the glass with ice. Top it off with sparkling water and enjoy.

FLAVOR BOOST: An ounce of tequila in this is also very good.

Per serving: Calories: 70; Total Fat: <1g; Saturated Fat: 0g; Protein: 1g; Total Carbohydrates: 17g; Fiber: 1g; Sugar: 12g; Cholesterol: 0mg

COCONUT-GINGER TONIC

SERVES: 2 **PREP TIME:** 5 minutes

This fancy drink helps with digestion, will help you sleep better, and will make you smarter, faster, stronger, and better in all aspects of your life. Okay . . . none of that is true, or maybe it is, who knows? It does taste good, though.

1 cup coconut water

2 teaspoons fresh lime juice

½ teaspoon grated fresh ginger

¼ teaspoon salt

1 cup crushed ice

1 cup tonic water

In a blender, combine the coconut water, lime juice, ginger, salt, and ice and blend until smooth. Divide the blended mix between two tall glasses and top with tonic water.

❋ FLAVOR BOOST: An ounce of gin or vodka makes this special drink even more special.

Per serving: Calories: 69; Total Fat: <1g; Saturated Fat: <1g; Protein: 1g; Total Carbohydrates: 17g; Fiber: 1g; Sugar: 14g; Cholesterol: 0mg

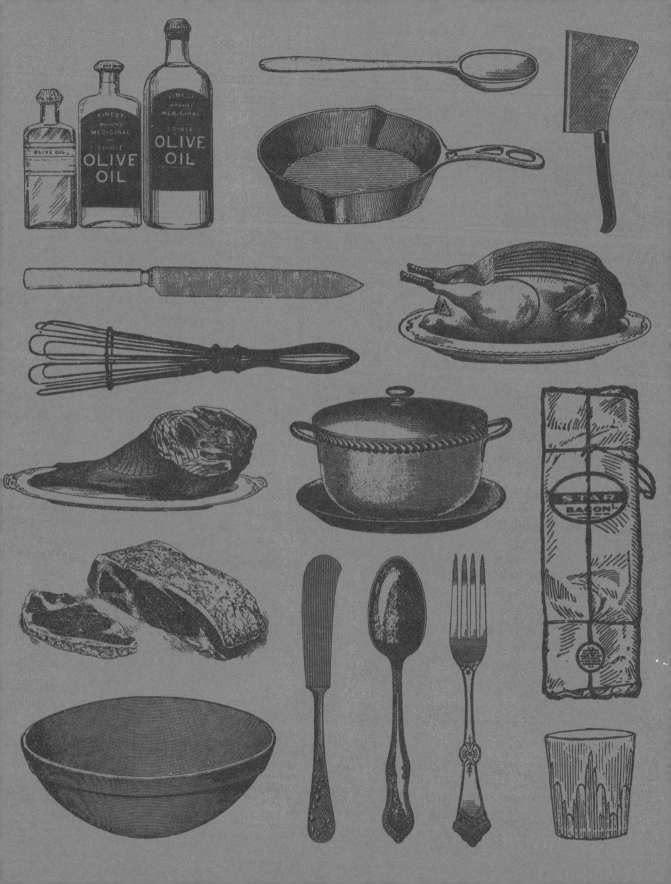

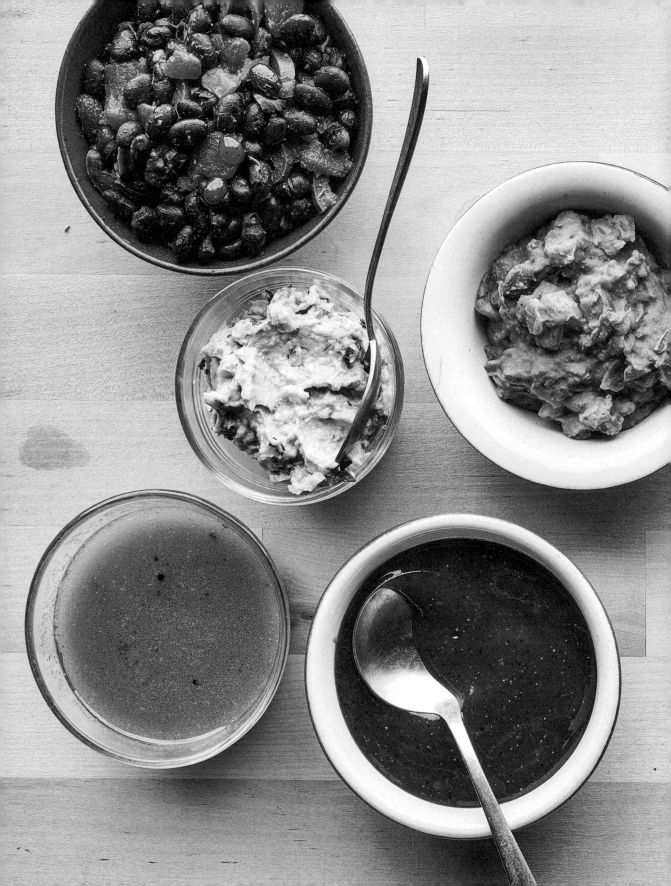

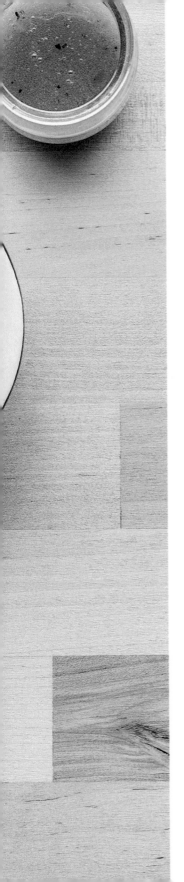

—10—

SUPERB SAUCES AND DRESSINGS

CREAMY AVOCADO-LIME DRESSING

(30) (DF) (x2) (GF) (OP) (VG)

MAKES: 1½ cups   **PREP TIME:** 5 minutes

This is a delicious multipurpose dressing that works just as well on a salad as it does on a spicy chicken sandwich. The creamy texture and fresh flavor will keep you coming back for more for years to come.

½ cup guacamole, homemade (page 48) or store-bought

½ cup mayonnaise

Juice of 1 lime

1 tablespoon sugar

¼ teaspoon chili powder

¼ teaspoon salt

⅛ teaspoon freshly ground black pepper

¼ cup water

In a medium bowl, whisk together the guacamole, mayonnaise, lime juice, sugar, chili powder, salt, and pepper. Whisk in enough of the water to thin the mixture until it just coats the back of a spoon.

 STORAGE TIP: Store in the fridge in an airtight container for up to 3 days.

Per serving (¼ cup): Calories: 147; Total Fat: 15g; Saturated Fat: 2g; Protein: <1g; Total Carbohydrates: 4g; Fiber: 1g; Sugar: 2g; Cholesterol: 8mg

BASIC VINAIGRETTE

MAKES: ¾ cup   **PREP TIME:** 5 minutes

As long as you keep the ratios in this basic vinaigrette the same, you can change the type of vinegar, the type of oil, and the ingredients you add. This means that you can make 75 percent of all salad dressings out there just because you know how to make this one. Yes, mind blown.

2 tablespoons red wine vinegar

1 tablespoon Dijon mustard

1 tablespoon honey

¼ teaspoon salt

¼ teaspoon freshly ground black pepper

½ cup olive oil

1. In a medium bowl, whisk together the vinegar, Dijon mustard, honey, salt, and pepper.

2. While whisking, add the oil very slowly. This is crucial, because if you add the oil all at once, the vinaigrette will fall apart. You need the mechanical agitation of whisking to break up the oil droplets so they can bond with the vinegar. Holy science, Batman!

3. After all the oil has been whisked in, continue to whisk it like crazy for about 30 seconds more.

✳ **STORAGE TIP:** Store the vinaigrette in the fridge in an airtight container for up to 1 month. Shake before serving.

Per serving (2 tablespoons): Calories: 173; Total Fat: 18g; Saturated Fat: 3g; Protein: <1g; Total Carbohydrates: 3g; Fiber: <1g; Sugar: 3g; Cholesterol: 0mg

SESAME-GINGER DRESSING

(30) (DF) (x2) (OP) (VG)

MAKES: ½ cup   **PREP TIME:** 5 minutes

The key ingredient to this salad dressing is toasted sesame oil. It can be found at most grocery stores in the international food section, or any Asian specialty grocery store. In addition to salad dressings, sesame oil is great in stir-fries or to flavor soups. This dressing also works well on chicken fingers or fish.

In a medium bowl, whisk together the vinegar, soy sauce, honey, ginger, and pepper. Slowly whisk in the sesame oil a few drops at a time until all of it has been incorporated.

STORAGE TIP: Store the dressing in the fridge in an airtight container for up to a month. Shake before serving.

2 tablespoons rice vinegar

1 tablespoon soy sauce

1 tablespoon honey

1 teaspoon grated fresh ginger

¼ teaspoon freshly ground black pepper

¼ cup sesame oil

Per serving (2 tablespoons): Calories: 141; Total Fat: 13g; Saturated Fat: 1.5g; Protein: 1g; Total Carbohydrates: 5g; Fiber: 1g; Sugar: 4g; Cholesterol: 0mg

CREAMY PESTO

MAKES: 1 cup   **PREP TIME:** 5 minutes

Classic pesto is a thing of beauty. It's simple to put together, has loads of flavor, and can be added to just about anything to give it a boost.

1 cup fresh basil leaves

½ cup olive oil

¼ cup pine nuts

2 tablespoons grated Parmesan cheese

¼ teaspoon salt

1. Pick off the stems at the ends of the basil leaves and discard. Wash the basil well and pat dry with a paper towel.

2. In a blender, combine the basil, olive oil, pine nuts, and Parmesan. Pulse the mixture until it's smooth and creamy. Stir the salt into the pesto.

✱ **STORAGE TIP:** You can store the pesto in the fridge in an airtight container for 3 or 4 days. Place a piece of plastic wrap on the surface of the pesto to help prevent it from oxidizing and turning black.

Per serving (¼ cup): Calories: 306; Total Fat: 33g; Saturated Fat: 5g; Protein: 2g; Total Carbohydrates: 2g; Fiber: 1g; Sugar: 1g; Cholesterol: 3mg

SIMPLE MARINARA SAUCE

SERVES: 4   **PREP TIME:** 5 minutes   **COOK TIME:** 25 minutes

This classic marinara sauce can be used as a pasta sauce or to braise meat or seafood. It can also be added to other dishes to enhance them or used as a pizza sauce. The simplicity of this recipe is deceiving because it does so much with so little. This is the kind of thing you should always have in your fridge.

1 (28-ounce) can whole peeled San Marzano tomatoes

¼ cup olive oil

½ cup diced onion

1 tablespoon minced garlic

1 tablespoon sugar

2 tablespoons chopped fresh basil

Salt

Freshly ground black pepper

1. Pour the tomatoes into a bowl and crush them into small pieces. Make sure to keep the tomatoes below the surface of the liquid when you squeeze them—this will prevent them from spraying everywhere.

2. Warm a large pot over medium heat. Add the olive oil and onion and cook for about 10 minutes, stirring every 1 to 2 minutes, until the onions turn a light brown.

3. Add the garlic and cook for 1 minute. Add the tomatoes and sugar and cook the sauce for 15 minutes to thicken and meld the flavors.

4. Remove from the heat, stir in the basil, and season with salt and pepper as needed.

※ SUBSTITUTION TIP: San Marzano tomatoes (which is a type of tomato and not a brand) are imported from Italy and have a superior taste to just about any canned tomatoes you will find here. But if you can't find them, buy the best quality tomatoes you can. Do not cheap out here: Because there are so few ingredients, the quality of the tomatoes is particularly important.

Per serving: Calories: 189; Total Fat: 14g; Saturated Fat: 2g; Protein: 2g; Total Carbohydrates: 13g; Fiber: 2g; Sugar: 9g; Cholesterol: 0mg

ALL-PURPOSE STIR-FRY SAUCE

MAKES: ¾ cup   **PREP TIME:** 5 minutes   **COOK TIME:** 10 minutes

Store-bought stir-fry sauces are loaded with stabilizers and preservatives that you can't pronounce. You can probably pronounce all the ingredients in this stir-fry sauce. This sauce is quick to make, stores well, and tastes delicious.

In a small bowl, mix the cornstarch and water. Add the cornstarch mixture to a medium pot along with the soy sauce, honey, sambal oelek, and ginger. Bring the pot to a boil, reduce the heat to low, and simmer it for 5 minutes.

✳ STORAGE TIP: Cool the sauce to room temperature, then store it in the refrigerator for up to 2 weeks in an airtight container.

2 teaspoons cornstarch

½ cup water

3 tablespoons soy sauce

1 tablespoon honey

2 teaspoons sambal oelek

1 tablespoon grated fresh ginger

Per serving (¼ cup): Calories: 38; Total Fat: <1g; Saturated Fat: 0g; Protein: 1g; Total Carbohydrates: 9g; Fiber: <1g; Sugar: 6g; Cholesterol: 0mg

ALL-PURPOSE BBQ SAUCE

MAKES: 2 cups   **PREP TIME:** 5 minutes   **COOK TIME:** 10 minutes

Every man should have his own special barbecue sauce recipe. This all-purpose barbecue sauce is a great sauce on its own, but it's also a solid starting point. Play around by adding different ingredients to create your signature BBQ sauce, then never tell anyone what's in it. Never. The first rule of barbecue sauce is that you don't talk about barbecue sauce.

---

1 cup ketchup

½ cup water

¼ cup packed light brown sugar

2 tablespoons apple cider vinegar

1 tablespoon yellow mustard

½ teaspoon freshly ground black pepper

¼ teaspoon cayenne pepper

¼ teaspoon salt

---

1. In a medium pot, whisk together the ketchup, water, brown sugar, vinegar, mustard, black pepper, cayenne, and salt. Bring to a boil over high heat, then reduce the heat to low and simmer, whisking for 5 minutes.

2. Remove from the heat. Let it cool slightly, then transfer to a mason jar or another heatproof, airtight container. Store in the fridge for up to 1 month.

✳ **FLAVOR BOOST:** Some ingredients you may consider adding are whiskey or beer, espresso, onion and garlic, or anything else you can think of.

Per serving (¼ cup): Calories: 49; Total Fat: <1g; Saturated Fat: 0g; Protein: <1g; Total Carbohydrates: 13g; Fiber: <1g; Sugar: 11g; Cholesterol: 0mg

BOURBON CARAMEL SAUCE

MAKES: 1 cup **PREP TIME:** 5 minutes **COOK TIME:** 15 minutes

What do you get when you carefully burn sugar then add bourbon to it? This bourbon caramel sauce. Okay, there's a little more to it than that, but not much more. This sauce is easy to make, tastes amazing, keeps in the fridge for a long time, and can be put on just about anything from bananas to ice cream.

½ **cup sugar**

¼ cup water

½ **cup heavy cream**

3 **tablespoons salted butter**

2 **tablespoons bourbon**

½ **teaspoon vanilla extract**

⅛ teaspoon salt

1. In a medium pot, combine the sugar and water and bring to a boil over high heat. Reduce the heat to medium-low and simmer the syrup for 7 to 10 minutes, until it starts to turn golden brown.

2. Once the syrup starts to turn golden brown, watch it very carefully. As soon as it turns caramel brown, add the cream into the pot and stir. Let the caramel boil for about 1 minute, then whisk in the butter little by little.

3. Remove from the heat and whisk in the bourbon, vanilla, and salt.

4. Let the sauce cool to room temperature, then transfer to a container and store in the refrigerator for up to 1 month. Heat slightly before using.

Per serving (¼ cup): Calories: 292; Total Fat: 19g; Saturated Fat: 12g; Protein: 1g; Total Carbohydrates: 26g; Fiber: 0g; Sugar: 26g; Cholesterol: 57mg

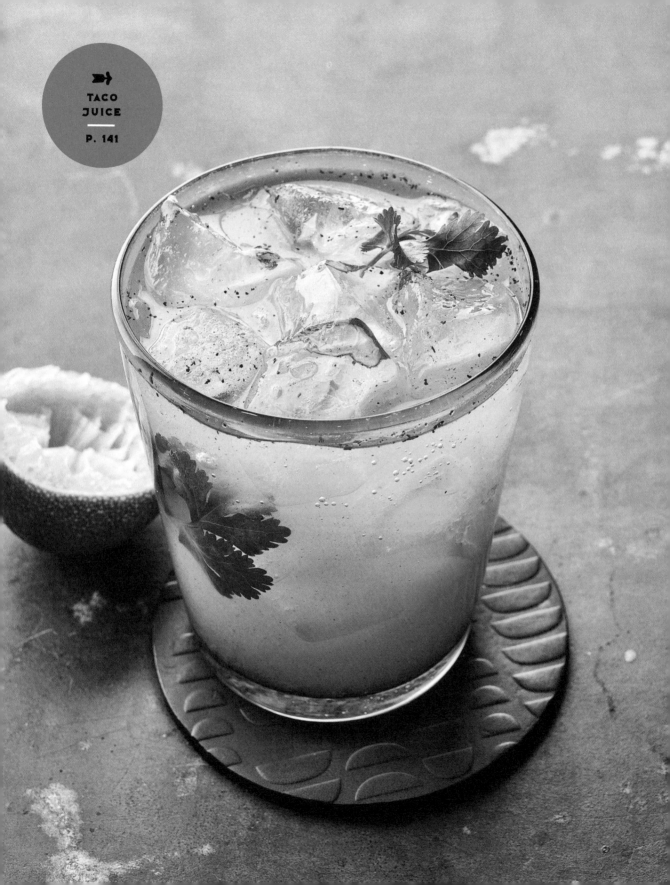

TACO
JUICE

P. 141

MEASUREMENT CONVERSIONS

	US STANDARD	US STANDARD (ounces)	METRIC (approximate)
VOLUME EQUIVALENTS *(Liquid)*	2 tablespoons	1 fl. oz.	30 mL
	¼ cup	2 fl. oz.	60 mL
	½ cup	4 fl. oz.	120 mL
	1 cup	8 fl. oz.	240 mL
	1½ cups	12 fl. oz.	355 mL
	2 cups or 1 pint	16 fl. oz.	475 mL
	4 cups or 1 quart	32 fl. oz.	1 L
	1 gallon	128 fl. oz.	4 L
VOLUME EQUIVALENTS *(Dry)*	⅛ teaspoon	————	0.5 mL
	¼ teaspoon	————	1 mL
	½ teaspoon	————	2 mL
	¾ teaspoon	————	4 mL
	1 teaspoon	————	5 mL
	1 tablespoon	————	15 mL
	¼ cup	————	59 mL
	⅓ cup	————	79 mL
	½ cup	————	118 mL
	⅔ cup	————	156 mL
	¾ cup	————	177 mL
	1 cup	————	235 mL
	2 cups or 1 pint	————	475 mL
	3 cups	————	700 mL
	4 cups or 1 quart	————	1 L
	½ gallon	————	2 L
	1 gallon	————	4 L
WEIGHT EQUIVALENTS	½ ounce	————	15 g
	1 ounce	————	30 g
	2 ounces	————	60 g
	4 ounces	————	115 g
	8 ounces	————	225 g
	12 ounces	————	340 g
	16 ounces or 1 pound	————	455 g

	FAHRENHEIT (F)	CELSIUS (C) (APPROXIMATE)
OVEN TEMPERATURES	250°F	120°C
	300°F	150°C
	325°F	180°C
	375°F	190°C
	400°F	200°C
	425°F	220°C
	450°F	230°C

INDEX

ACKNOWLEDGMENTS

This book would not be possible without the love and support of my mom, Linda; my wife, Suzanne; my son, Llewyn; and the rest of my family and friends. Nor without the encouragement and guidance from my former chefs, mentors, and colleagues. Thank you to all of you who have pushed, helped, and guided me throughout the years. And to everyone at Callisto Media, without whom this book would not exist. A special thank you to The Baketones, Dr. Emily Kirk, Evan Fougere, and Brad Wammes.

ABOUT THE AUTHOR

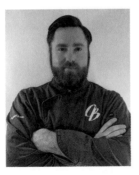

BENJAMIN KELLY is a Red Seal chef and blogger from Nova Scotia, Canada. For more than 20 years he has worked in a wide variety of restaurants from Canada's east coast to its far north.

Ben's love of food first developed as a young child cooking corn chowder and shepherd's pie alongside his mother. That love grew as Ben was guided through his culinary journey by numerous chefs and teachers. Ben's passion now extends to teaching anyone who wants to learn about food and how to cook.

Today Ben owns and operates a personal chef service and catering company as well as a successful food blog called Chef's Notes (ChefsNotes.com). You can find him on social media @chefbenkelly.